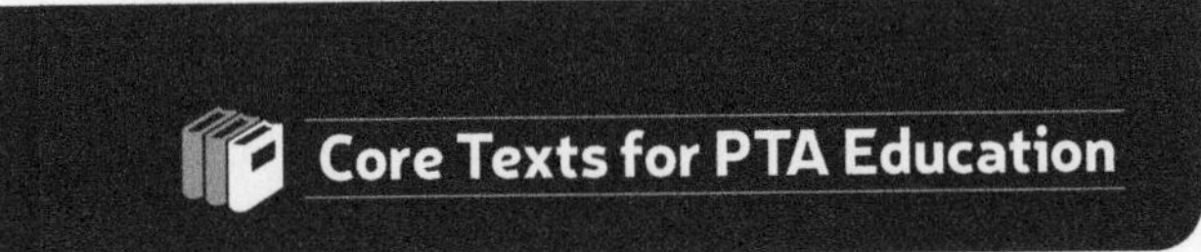

Documentation Basics for the Physical Therapist Assistant

Third Edition

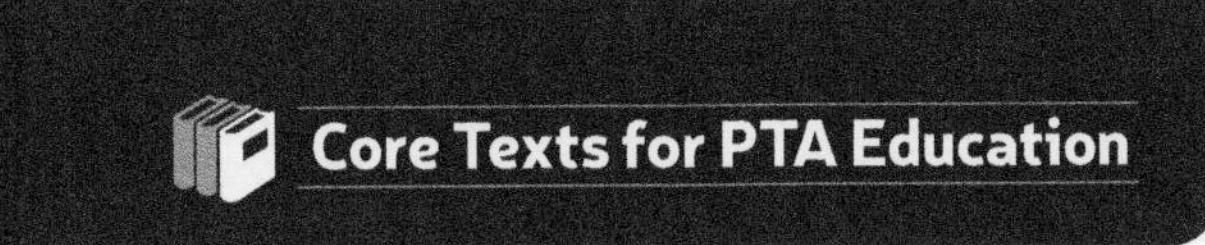

Documentation Basics for the Physical Therapist Assistant

Third Edition

MIA L. ERICKSON, PT, EdD, CHT, ATC
Midwestern University
Physical Therapy Department
Glendale, AZ

REBECCA MCKNIGHT, PT, MS
Educational Consultant
Reach Consulting, LLC
Forsyth, MO

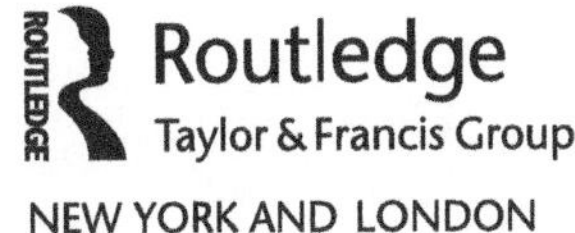

NEW YORK AND LONDON

Instructors: *Documentation Basics for the Physical Therapist Assistant, Third Edition* Instructor's Manual is also available. Don't miss this important companion to *Documentation Basics for the Physical Therapist Assistant, Third Edition.* To obtain the Instructor's Manual, please visit www.routledge.com/9781630914028

First published 2018 by SLACK Incorporated

Published 2024 by Routledge
605 Third Avenue, New York, NY 10158

and by Routledge
4 Park Square, Milton Park, Abingdon, Oxon OX14 4RN

Routledge is an imprint of the Taylor & Francis Group, an informa business

Dr. Mia L. Erickson and Rebecca McKnight *have no financial or proprietary interest in the materials presented herein.*

Names: Erickson, Mia L., editor. | McKnight, Rebecca, 1969- editor. |
Preceded by (work): Erickson, Mia L. Documentation basics.
Title: Documentation basics for the physical therapist assistant / edited by
Mia L. Erickson, Rebecca McKnight.
Description: Third edition. | Thorofare, NJ : SLACK Incorporated, [2018] |
Preceded by Documentation basics / Mia L. Erickson, Rebecca McKnight. 2nd
ed. 2012. | Includes bibliographical references and index.
Identifiers: LCCN 2017054078 | ISBN 9781630914028 (pbk.) |
Subjects: | MESH: Physical Therapy Specialty--organization & administration |
Medical Records | Physical Therapist Assistants
Classification: LCC RM705 | NLM WB 460 | DDC 615.8/2023--dc23 LC record available at https://lccn.loc.gov/2017054078

ISBN: 9781630914028 (pbk)
ISBN: 9781003523871 (ebk)

DOI: 10.4324/9781003523871

Contents

Contents

About the Authors

Mia L. Erickson, PT, EdD, CHT, ATC, is a faculty member in the Physical Therapy Department at Midwestern University in Glendale, AZ. Mia earned a bachelor's degree from West Virginia University in secondary education in 1994 and a master of science degree in physical therapy from the University of Indianapolis in 1996. Mia earned a doctoral degree in education from West Virginia University with an emphasis on curriculum and instruction in 2002. Her clinical practice is in the area of hand and upper-extremity rehabilitation.

Rebecca McKnight, PT, MS, received her bachelor of science degree in physical therapy from St. Louis University in 1992 and her postprofessional master of science degree from Rocky Mountain University of Health Professions in 1999. She taught at Ozarks Technical Community College for 14 years, serving as Program Director for 9 of those years. Rebecca is an active member of the American Physical Therapy Association and is a former chair of the Physical Therapist Assistant Educators Special Interest Group of the education section. Rebecca has spoken at many national meetings on physical therapist assistant curriculum design and programmatic assessment. She is the 2009 recipient of the F.A. Davis Award for Outstanding Physical Therapist Assistant Educator. Rebecca has been providing educational consultation in the areas of curriculum design, development, and assessment for physical therapist assistant programs nationwide since 2007.

Preface

We would like to thank you for choosing the Third Edition of *Documentation Basics for the Physical Therapist Assistant*. We think that you will find some substantial changes that make this edition more modern, reflecting contemporary principles in documentation. Two of the biggest changes are incorporation of the *International Classification of Functioning, Disability and Health* (ICF) disablement model (vs other models that have been discussed in previous editions) and further integration of the electronic medical record. The ICF serves as the framework for several important aspects of this text. Throughout, we encourage readers to really think about disablement and disablement concepts when writing notes. This includes documenting impairments in body structure and function in addition to activity limitations and participation restriction. We also encourage the reader to frequently note improvements in impairments, activity limitations, and participation restrictions brought on by the intervention provided in objective terms so that others reading the documentation can see the improvement.

This edition has been updated in its discussion of the electronic medical record. In addition to describing the differences in documentation methods using a computer vs a paper chart, this edition features a stand-alone chapter on the electronic medical record. It walks the reader through differences in the electronic health and medical records and discusses the rationale for change to electronic record keeping. The book also incorporates some evidence tied to benefits and challenges of computerized documentation. We were fortunate enough to have WebPT® (Phoenix, AZ) allow us to integrate screen shots from its computerized documentation system. This enables the reader to see what a screen would look like in various parts of the medical record.

We continue to incorporate concepts related to documenting the rationale for treatment and note how the unique skills of the physical therapist assistant were used in patient management. Examples, or "how-tos," are also provided. We feel like these changes are unique to our text and can help readers to understand these important aspects of documentation in today's payer system.

While we continue our instruction in writing a note using the SOAP (subjective, objective, assessment, and plan) structure, we recognize and point out its flaws. We still believe that understanding parts of notes using the SOAP acronym can help students to learn the fundamentals and then, when they get to the clinical site, they can integrate their knowledge into the software or charting system used at that site.

Again, we are happy to provide you with this updated version of our book, and we hope that you enjoy it, whether you are using it as a physical therapist assistant student, a physical therapist assistant educator, or a clinician.

Preface

Chapter 1

Disablement and Physical Therapy Documentation

Mia L. Erickson, PT, EdD, CHT, ATC

KEY TERMS Activity | Activity limitation | American Physical Therapy Association | Biomedical model | Body functions | Body structures | Contextual factor | Disablement | Documentation | Environmental factor | *International Classification of Functioning, Disability and Health* | *International Classification of Diseases, Tenth Revision* | Participation | Participation restriction | Personal factor | Physical therapist

KEY ABBREVIATIONS APTA | ICD-10 | ICF | PT | WHO

Chapter Objectives

After reading this chapter, the reader will be able to do the following:

1. Define disablement.
2. Define terminology used in the *International Classification of Functioning, Disability and Health* (ICF).
3. Differentiate between impairment, activity limitation, and participation restriction.
4. Define documentation.
5. Describe the need for common language in physical therapy documentation.
6. Describe how disablement concepts can be integrated into physical therapy documentation.

A traditional approach to defining a person's health comes from the biomedical model in which health means free or absent from disease.[1] The biomedical model implies that accurate diagnosis and identification of the patient's biological defects can directly lead to selection of interventions that will maximize health outcomes.[1] In this model, however, there is little emphasis on how the disease affects the person's ability to function or participate within society on a daily basis. Over the last few decades, many rehabilitation professionals have shifted their focus away from managing the disease or pathology and have moved toward managing the consequences of the disease or condition. It has become more common to focus on these consequences as they pertain to the individual's ability to carry out tasks and function within society. Assessing functional performance and describing functional status are now primary components of the physical therapist's examination of the patient. Verbrugge and Jette[2] described the consequences that chronic and acute conditions have on specific body system function and on a person's ability to act in necessary, usual, expected, and personally desired ways in his or her society as disablement. These authors explained that disablement is a "process," indicating that it is dynamic, or a trajectory of functional consequences over time. A more contemporary approach to physical therapy patient management is to incorporate disablement and disablement concepts.

Individuals and groups throughout the world have developed disablement frameworks. Disablement frameworks are useful for providing a common language for health care providers, and they can serve as a basic archi-

Erickson ML, McKnight R. *Documentation Basics for the Physical Therapist Assistant, Third Edition* (pp. 1-7)

Example 1-1

The following definitions have been endorsed by the World Health Organization as part of the ICF[3]:

- **Functioning** is an umbrella term that includes all body functions, activities, and participation.
- **Disability** serves as an umbrella term for dysfunction at any one or more of the following levels: impairment, activity limitation, and participation restriction.
- **Body functions** are physiological functions of the body (including psychological function).
- **Body structures** are anatomical bodily structures, such as organs and limbs.
- **Impairments** are problems with body functions (physiological, psychological) or structures, such as a deviation or loss.
- **Activity** is the execution of a task or activity by an individual.
- **Activity limitations** are difficulties that might be encountered by an individual who is attempting to complete a task or carry out an activity.
- **Participation** is involvement in a life situation, such as work or school.
- **Participation restrictions** are problems an individual might face while involved in life situations.
- **Contextual factors** are the complete factors that make up a person's life and living, including his or her background.
- **Environmental factors** are the physical, social, and attitudinal environmental in which people live and carry out their lives. These include things immediate to the individual, such as his or her home or workplace, and the larger social context, such as government agencies designed to assist people with disabilities.
- **Personal factors** are factors specific to the individual and his or her background. These include things such as age, gender, social habits, health habits, upbringing, and coping strategies.

tecture for research, policy, and clinical care.[2] In addition to providing infrastructure, disablement frameworks define health in terms that go beyond the patient's medical diagnosis or disease, acknowledging the importance of societal, psychological, and physical functioning. Rather than placing the measure of health on the disease process itself, these models have helped providers to shift toward understanding an individual's ability to carry out necessary life tasks and to function within society. Disablement frameworks have attempted to delineate a pathway from pathology to functional outcome while recognizing the social, psychological, and environmental factors that can facilitate or interfere with the pathway.[2] The purpose of this chapter is to introduce you to the disablement framework used in physical therapy practice and to introduce the purpose of using disablement and disablement concepts in clinical documentation.

International Classification of Functioning, Disability and Health

The ICF, originally known as the *International Classification of Impairments, Disabilities, and Handicaps*, was endorsed by the 54th World Health Assembly and released in 2001. The ICF provides a uniform, standard language for describing an individual's health and health-related state that moves beyond his or her diagnosis.[3] In 2008, the American Physical Therapy Association (APTA) House of Delegates voted to endorse the ICF and, as a result, APTA publications, documents, and communications have been updated to incorporate the ICF language (Example 1-1).[4] Therefore, the ICF serves to provide a common language for physical therapists to communicate.

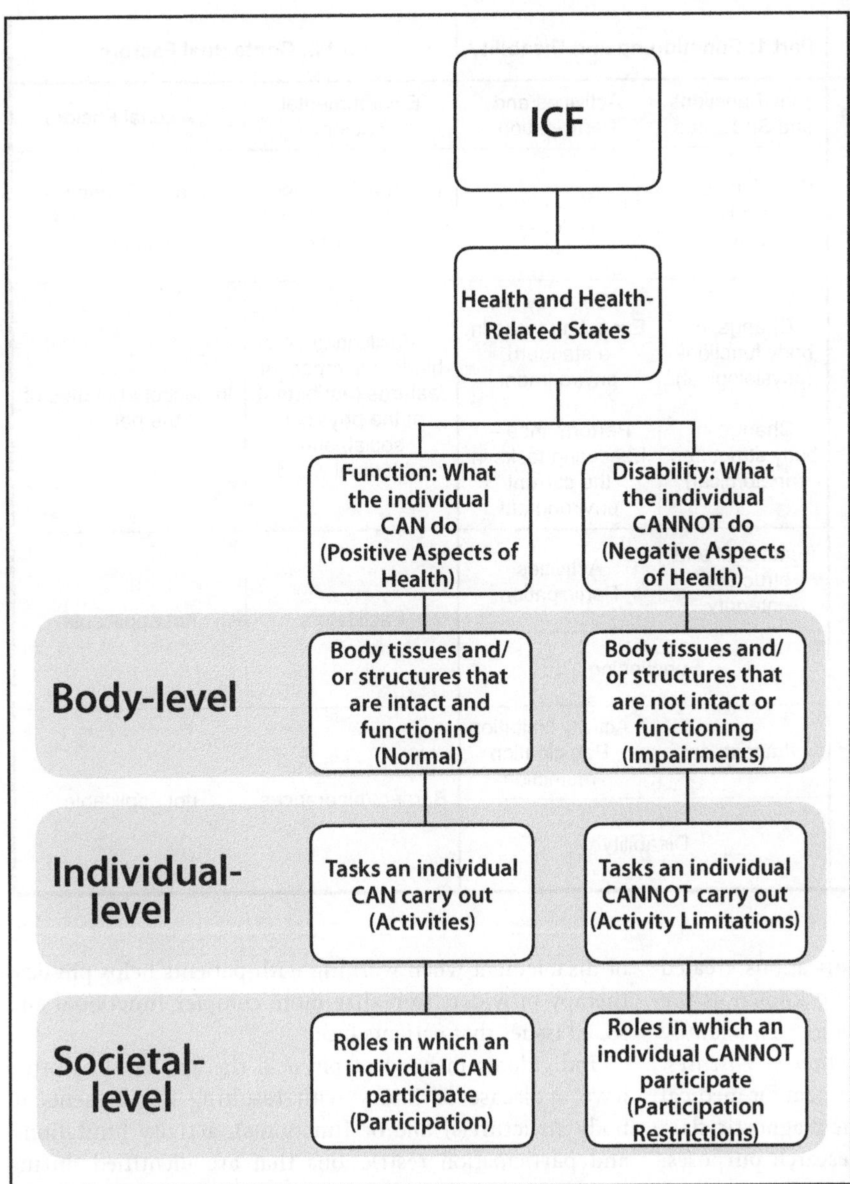

Figure 1-1. Overview of the *International Classification of Functioning, Disability and Health*.[3] The string of boxes on the left represents the positive aspects of the health state or condition. The string of boxes on the right represents deviations from normal, or the negative aspects of health.

In the ICF, the individual's health or health-related state is described in terms of function and disability. What the individual can do is known as functioning, or the positive aspects of health. What the individual cannot do is known as disability, or the negative aspects of health (Figure 1-1).[3] Function and disability comprise Part 1 of the ICF. Part 1 is further divided into the following 2 components: (1) body functions (physiological function) and body structures (anatomical structures) and (2) activities and participation (Figure 1-2).[3] In categorizing an individual's health according to the ICF, a health care provider would describe body structures and functions that are intact and those that are not intact. Any deviation(s) from normal body structure and/or function are known as impairments. For the activities and participation component, the examiner identifies functional tasks that the individual can do (known as activities) and those that he or she cannot do (known as activity limitations). The examiner also identifies life roles that the individual can carry out (known as participation) and those that he or she cannot carry out (known as participation restrictions; see Figure 1-1).[3]

The ICF also accounts for contextual factors that might facilitate or impede the patient's function. These appear in Part 2, which also includes environmental and personal factors that affect the individual's functioning and disability. Environmental factors are external factors that are either within the individual's immediate environment or part of a larger social structure and that affect the individual's ability to participate in society. These might be facilitators, which enhance participation, or barriers, which deter participation. Environmental factors include things such as physical structures (eg, ramps, stairs, curbs). Personal factors are those that are unique to the individual, such as attitude, mood, or family support (see Figure 1-2).[3]

Figure 1-2. The *International Classification of Functioning, Disability and Health*[3] from the WHO. (Reprinted with permission from the WHO.)

	Part 1: Functioning and Disability		Part 2: Contextual Factors	
Components	Body Functions and Structures	Activities and Participation	Environmental Factors	Personal Factors
Domains	Body functions Body structures	Life areas (tasks, actions)	External influences on functioning and disability	Internal influences on functioning and disability
Constructs	Change in body functions (physiological) Change in body structures (anatomical)	Capacity -- Executing tasks in a standard environment Performance -- Executing tasks in the current environment	Facilitating or hindering impact of features (attributes) of the physical, social, and attitudinal world	Impact of attributes of the person
Positive aspect	Functional and structural integrity	Activities Participation	Facilitators	not applicable
	Functioning			
Negative aspect	Impairment	Activity limitation Participation restriction	Barriers/hindrances	not applicable
	Disability			

The ICF is part of a "family" of classifications created by the World Health Organization (WHO) known as the WHO *Family of International Classifications.*[5] This family also includes the *International Classification of Diseases, Tenth Revision* (ICD-10), a classification system for medical diagnoses and diseases. The ICD-10 is the diagnostic classification standard for all clinical and research purposes. It defines the universe of disease, disorders, injuries, and other related health conditions, listed in a comprehensive format.[6] The ICF and ICD-10 are meant to complement each other in that the ICD-10 provides a catalog of medical diagnoses, diseases, disorders, and health conditions and the ICF provides corresponding information on function and disability. Used together, they provide a broader picture of an individual's health.[7]

Physical Therapy and Disablement

The ICF provides clinicians with standardized terminology and a framework to aid in exploring the impact of disease or injury on an individual's daily life. More specifically, physical therapy providers can use the ICF to help understand the consequences of the disease or condition on the body systems and the impact on the individual's activity level and participation within society. Consideration of disablement when working with patients helps physical therapy providers to realize more complex functional and social issues that patients face.

Individuals in need of physical therapy services often have a disease or injury with resulting impairments in body structure(s) and/or function(s), activity limitations, and participation restrictions that are identified during the physical therapist's examination. Impairments can be limitations in range of motion, strength, endurance, or balance, to name a few. But to see how the patient's ability to participate in society has been compromised, the examination must go beyond the impairment level. It is our responsibility to understand how impairments affect the patient's day-to-day activities and participation in a variety of settings and situations; therefore, the physical therapist's examination of patient function includes assessment of the following: (1) activities such as bed mobility, transfers, hygiene, self-care, and home management (eg, yardwork, household cleaning); and (2) participation such as the ability to work, go to school, play, and participate in community activities (eg, going to the grocery store or bank). By understanding an individual's impairments and his or her activity limitations and participation restrictions, we can better understand the degree of disability associated with the pathology for the individual patient.

Documentation and Disablement

Documentation, otherwise known as medical record keeping, has been defined as "any entry into the individual's health record, such as a(n) consultation reports, initial examination reports, progress notes, flow sheets, checklists, re-examination reports, or summations of care, that identifies the care or services and the individual's response to intervention."[8] Complete documentation also includes the physician prescription(s) and certification(s), communication with other care providers, copies of exercise programs or patient instructions, and any other disciplines' notes or comments that support the interventions.[9]

As you will read in subsequent chapters, documentation will serve many purposes, but, regardless of the purpose, your documentation should reflect disablement. One reason for integrating disablement concepts in physical therapy documentation is to achieve consistency in terminology because our notes are the sole record of the episode of care provided to each patient or client. Another reason is to show the reader how the patient's pathology and impairments influence his or her activities and participation in daily life. Disablement concepts serve as a foundation for this text. Throughout the chapters, you will be reminded of the following 3 important disablement concepts that should be integrated into your clinical documentation:

1. Documentation should reflect not only measures of impairment, but also measures of activity limitations and participation restrictions.
2. Documentation should describe how the patient's impairments relate or contribute to his or her activity limitations and participation restrictions.
3. Documentation should explain how physical therapy interventions are bringing about changes in impairments, activity limitations, and participation restrictions that relate to the patient's therapy goals.

References

1. MacDermid JC, Law M, Michlovitz SL. Outcome measurement in evidence-based rehabilitation. In: Law M, MacDermid JC, eds. *Evidence-Based Rehabilitation: A Guide to Practice. 3rd ed.* Thorofare, NJ: SLACK Incorporated; 2014:65-104.
2. Verbrugge LM, Jette AM. The disablement process. *Soc Sci Med.* 1994;38(1):1-14.
3. World Health Organization. *International Classification of Functioning, Disability and Health*: ICF. Geneva: World Health Organization; 2001.
4. American Physical Therapy Association. *International Classification of Functioning, Disability, and Health.* APTA Website. http://www.apta.org/ICF/. Updated August 23, 2013. Accessed October 24, 2016.
5. Madden R, Sykes C, Ustun TB. *World Health Organization Family of International Classifications: definition, scope, and purpose.* World Health Organization Website. http://www.who.int/classifications/en/FamilyDocument2007.pdf?ua=1. Updated February 2, 2012. Accessed October 24, 2016.
6. World Health Organization. *Classifications: International Classification of Disease.* WHO Website. http://www.who.int/classifications/icd/en/. Updated June 29, 2016. Accessed October 24, 2016.
7. Escorpizo R, Bemis-Dougherty A. Introduction to special issue: a review of the International Classification of Functioning, Disability and Health and physical therapy over the years. *Physiother Res Int.* 2015;20(4):200-209.
8. American Physical Therapy Association. *Guide to Physical Therapist Practice 3.0.* APTA Website. http://guidetoptpractice.apta.org/content/1/SEC2.body. Updated August 1, 2014. Accessed October 24, 2016.
9. Redgate N, Foto M. Pay by the rules: avoid Medicare audits and reduce payment denials with a sound strategy and proper documentation. *Physical Therapy Products.* 2003;October/November:28-30.

Review Questions

1. How is a person's health determined today as opposed to 5 decades ago?

2. In your own words, describe disablement.

3. According to the ICF, what is the difference between an impairment, an activity limitation, and a participation restriction?

4. Why is there a need for disablement models today? Why are they important to you?

5. What is physical therapy documentation? What does it include?

6. Give some examples of ways a physical therapist assistant can incorporate disablement concepts into his or her documentation.

7. Look at the examples below. Determine if each would be considered an impairment in body function or structure, an activity limitation, or a participation restriction.
   __________ Taking a bath
   __________ Going to school
   __________ Brushing teeth
   __________ Limited shoulder motion
   __________ Walking in the community
   __________ Going to the grocery store
   __________ Ascending/descending stairs
   __________ Turning a door knob
   __________ Poor endurance
   __________ Writing
   __________ Working
   __________ Poor balance
   __________ Donning socks
   __________ Bathing

Read the following scenarios and identify the impairments, activity limitations and participation restrictions.

8. You are working with a 70-year-old male who had a total hip replacement 3 weeks ago. He is now able to move in and out of the bed independently, transfer to a chair placed at the bedside, and ambulate 25 feet with a standard walker. He wants to return to driving, golfing, and playing with his grandchildren.

9. You are working with a 10-year-old female in the school system. Her medical diagnosis (pathology) is spastic diplegia cerebral palsy. You have been working on ambulating up and down the stairs (which she can perform with minimum assist of 1, a quad cane, and a handrail) and increasing the speed of her gait. At the present time, she leaves her classes early so that she can make it to the next one on time, and she uses the elevator rather than the stairs.

10. Your patient is a 15-year-old who sustained a traumatic closed head injury in a motorcycle accident. He is confused and disoriented, and he requires constant supervision for his safety. He can walk and get in and out of bed with supervision. He can also ascend and descend stairs with supervision. He is unable to work.

Chapter 2

The Physical Therapy Episode of Care

Rebecca McKnight, PT, MS

KEY TERMS Diagnosis | Episode of care | Evaluation | Examination | Intervention | Outcome | Patient/client management | Plan of care | Prognosis

Chapter Objectives

After reading this chapter, the reader will be able to do the following:

1. Describe a physical therapy episode of care from point of entry to discontinuation of services.
2. Discuss the various ways patients access a physical therapist for care.
3. List the 6 elements of the Patient/Client Management Model.
4. Define and describe each of the 6 elements of the Patient/Client Management Model.
5. Discuss the roles of the physical therapist and physical therapist assistant within the Patient/Client Management Model.
6. Describe the physical therapist assistant's responsibilities related to patient care, documentation, and communication.

Sadie had come to terms with the fact that she has multiple sclerosis. After all, she had witnessed her aunt Linda, who also was diagnosed with multiple sclerosis, living a fruitful and productive life even though she had to make some changes in her daily routine. This did not, however, keep Sadie from getting frustrated with some of the new issues she had to face. Most recently, she had been experiencing fatigue, which had been hindering her ability to function at work. Even more frustrating than the fatigue were the new symptoms of clumsiness affecting her arms and legs and causing her difficulty with most of her activities. Upon her neurologist's suggestion, Sadie had been admitted to the local hospital for treatment. After returning home from the hospital, Sadie was still experiencing difficulties with her daily tasks. Her neurologist recommended that Sadie seek a physical therapist to address her coordination and balance issues. Sadie sat in front of her computer with a list of physical therapists in the area and began to research each physical therapist to see whether any had experience with working with individuals with her problems.

To actively participate in the provision of physical therapy services efficiently and with confidence, you must start with an understanding of the entire physical therapy care process. This will enable you to appreciate the role that you will play in the provision of interventions and the role of your supervising physical therapist(s). Based upon this understanding, you will begin to grasp how integral communication is to the entire process and how essential effective documentation is in ensuring that patients

Erickson ML, McKnight R. *Documentation Basics for the Physical Therapist Assistant, Third Edition* (pp. 9-18)

"receive appropriate, comprehensive, efficient, and effective quality care."[1] This chapter examines how patients access physical therapy services. We provide a general outline of components of physical therapy care throughout an episode of care. We then take a close look at the American Physical Therapy Association (APTA) Patient/Client Management Model and the roles of the physical therapist and physical therapist assistant within the components of the model. Finally, we touch on the relationship between the Patient/Client Management Model and documentation, providing the foundation for upcoming chapters.

Physical Therapist Services

The APTA *Guide to Physical Therapist Practice*[1] outlines the physical therapy process by means of the Patient/Client Management Model. This model defines and describes 6 elements required to ensure that optimal physical therapy care occurs during a patient's episode of care. These essential components include examination, evaluation, diagnosis, prognosis, intervention, and outcomes (Table 2-1)[1]. We will look at each of these components in more detail, but first we need to consider how patients/clients access a physical therapist to receive care.

Patient Point of Entry

Individuals enter physical therapy care by either self-referral or when referred by another health care practitioner. Self-referral, also known as direct access, is when an individual seeks care from a physical therapist without first obtaining a referral from another primary care provider, such as a physician. Currently, all state practice acts allow a physical therapist to perform an evaluation and provide some form of treatment without a physician referral.[2] However, most states still have restrictions that limit what care the physical therapist can provide in the absence of meeting additional conditions. As of June 2016, only 18 states allow unrestricted access to physical therapy services. Unrestricted access is when there are no legal restrictions or additional conditions required of a physical therapist to provide all aspects of patient/client management. The level of patient access to physical therapy services and types of restrictions per state law can be viewed in the APTA document *Levels of Patient Access to Physical Therapist Services in the States*: http://www.apta.org/uploadedFiles/APTAorg/Advocacy/State/Issues/Direct_Access/DirectAccessbyState.pdf.

In addition to self-referral, patients access a physical therapist when referred by another health care provider. Depending on state regulations, physical therapists can receive referrals from physicians, physician assistants, chiropractors, nurse practitioners, midwives, and dentists. Often, patients initially access physical therapy services during a hospitalization for disease or injury. At other times, individuals will enter physical therapy care through outpatient services, home health services, or school-based services.

The Patient/Client Management Model

Once an individual has accessed a physical therapist, the therapist will initiate the episode of care through the examination/evaluation process. This process must be initiated prior to the provision of any interventions. During the examination, the physical therapist collects data that will be used in determining appropriate management strategies. The mental process of analyzing the data and making clinical decisions based upon the information is referred to as the evaluation. As part of the evaluation, the physical therapist will determine a physical therapy diagnosis, the patient's prognosis for achieving expected outcomes, and what intervention strategies will be implemented. Once interventions are initiated, the physical therapist will monitor the patient's progress through a review of his or her outcomes. Let's take a closer look at these elements.

Examination

As indicated above, the purpose of the examination is for the physical therapist to collect data to guide clinical decision making. An examination consists of the following 3 components: (1) history, (2) systems review, and (3) tests and measures. Patient history can be obtained from the patient or the patient's caregiver, family, other individuals familiar with the patient's history (eg, other health care providers, case managers, teachers, employers, significant others),[1] and medical record if one is available. History data include information related to several areas, including the current condition for which the individual is seeking physical therapy services and current or past health information (Sidebar 2-1). Additionally, the physical therapist will ask about the patient's home situation, support system, and community involvement. Patient history data allow the therapist to gain a holistic view of the individual and help to contextualize the patient's reason for seeking physical therapy services. The information is essential for the physical therapist to consider when determining the patient's prognosis.

After obtaining a picture of the patient's condition and concerns through history taking, the physical therapist performs a systems review. A systems review is a "hands-on examination" where the therapist performs limited examination of the patient's overall medical health by reviewing the patient's cardiovascular/pulmonary system, integumentary system, musculoskeletal system, neuromuscular system, communication ability, affect, cognition, language, and learning style.[3] Based on information gathered during the history and systems review, the physical therapist will select and perform appropriate tests and measures.[1] Tests and measures are methods and techniques that the

Table 2-1[1]

Elements of the Patient/Client Management Model

Element	Who/When	Includes	Source of Information	Purpose
Examination	Performed by the physical therapist on all patients prior to provision of interventions	• History • Systems review • Tests and measures	• Medical record review • Patient interview • Communication with others	Provides data needed for the physical therapist to determine the plan of care
Evaluation	Performed by the physical therapist in conjunction with, and based upon, the examination	• Plan of care (goals and interventions to be provided) • Involvement of other providers	The clinical judgement of the physical therapist based upon findings from the examination	Allows others (including the physical therapist assistant) insight into the anticipated level of improvement, intervention plan, and frequency and duration of services
Diagnosis	Determined by the physical therapist	A label which describes the dysfunction requiring physical therapist interventions		
Prognosis	Determined by the physical therapist	The predicted level of improvement, treatment goals, expected outcomes, duration and frequency of treatment and interventions to be used		
Intervention	Done by the physical therapist or physical therapist assistant (as directed) to produce the changes in the patient's condition	• Patient or client instruction • Airway clearance techniques • Assistive technology • Biophysical agents • Functional training in self-care and domestic, work, community, social, and civic life • Integumentary repair and protection techniques • Manual therapy techniques • Motor function	Specific interventions to be provided per the categories outlined by the physical therapist in the plan of care	Decrease inflammation, decrease pain, increase motion, improve functional abilities, etc
Outcomes	Performed by the physical therapist or the physical therapist assistant	Tests and observations consistent with initial examination	Initial examination and follow-up documentation	Used to determine patient response to interventions and progress toward goals

Sidebar 2-1

Categories of Information Gathered in History Portion of the Examination

- Activities and participation
- Current condition(s)/chief complaint(s)
- Employment/work (eg, job, school, play)
- Family history
- Functional status and activity level
- Health restoration and prevention needs
- General demographics (eg, age, sex, race)
- General health status
- Growth and development
- Living environment
- Medical/surgical history
- Medications
- Systems review via medical chart review including other clinical tests
- Social history
- Social/health habits (past and current)

Sidebar 2-2

Categories of Tests and Measures Used by Physical Therapists

- Aerobic capacity/endurance
- Anthropometric characteristics
- Assistive technology
- Balance
- Circulation
- Community, social, and civic life
- Cranial and peripheral nerve integrity
- Education life
- Environmental factors
- Gait
- Integumentary integrity
- Joint integrity and mobility
- Mental functions
- Mobility
- Motor function
- Muscle performance
- Neuromotor development and sensory processing
- Pain
- Posture
- Range of motion
- Reflex integrity
- Self-care and domestic life
- Sensory integrity
- Skeletal integrity
- Ventilation and respiration
- Work life

therapist uses to gather data needed to determine the diagnosis and prognosis and to guide clinical decision making (Sidebar 2-2). Tests and measures are also used later in patient/client management to evaluate outcomes and to note patient progression.

Evaluation

The physical therapist analyzes the information gathered during the examination process and makes clinical judgments about the findings. This clinical decision-making process is known as the evaluation. Evaluation is a continuous process. It begins with the first data gathered during the history taking and undergirds all decisions made throughout the entire episode of care; however, as a component of initiation of care, evaluation is the process that the physical therapist utilizes to determine a physical therapy diagnosis and prognosis and to establish the plan of care.

Clinical decisions made by the physical therapist include whether to initiate physical therapy care and whether there is a need for other health care provider involvement. The involvement of other health care providers can include referral, consultation, comanagement, or a combination of these. A physical therapist will choose to refer a patient when the patient's condition requires the management of a different health care provider. This might be because the patient has a condition that falls outside of the scope of practice of the physical therapist or it could be because the patient's physical therapy needs fall outside of the physical therapist's personal scope of practice (knowledge, abilities, or experience). The following are examples of each situation:

- Outside of a physical therapist's scope of practice
  - *During the examination, the physical therapist notes findings consistent with congestive heart failure. The therapist refers the patient to a cardiologist so the patient can receive the necessary medical care.*

- Outside of a physical therapist's personal scope of practice
    - *A physical therapist's examination reveals a vestibular disorder. Although interventions for vestibular disorders fall within the physical therapy scope of practice, the therapist is aware of another therapist in the area who specializes in vestibular disorder therapy and, therefore, refers the patient to ensure that he or she receives optimal care.*

Even when the physical therapist chooses to refer a patient to another care provider for services, the physical therapist is still obligated to determine whether the patient is appropriate for care and, in both scenarios above, it is possible that the therapist might retain some patient care management responsibilities. In the scenario with the patient referred to the cardiologist, the physical therapist might choose to work with the patient on energy conservation techniques and modified activities of daily living while waiting for the cardiologist report. In the second scenario, the patient might also have other physical therapy problems for which the initiating physical therapist has more experience and is a more-qualified professional to address. In this case, the therapists would divide the patient management based on their levels of expertise and should closely collaborate. This would be an example of comanagement described below.

In some cases, the physical therapist may choose to retain care of the patient but consult with another provider due to the nature of the condition. Examples of other providers with whom the physical therapist might consult include a physician, a dentist, a nurse practitioner, a psychologist, an occupational therapist, or even another physical therapist. It is appropriate for the physical therapist to seek the advice of any provider who can provide insight that would be beneficial to the patient. The following are 2 examples of incidents when a physical therapist consults with another provider:

- A physical therapist consults with another discipline.
    - *A physical therapist is working with a patient with long-term activity limitations and participation restrictions due to a cerebrovascular accident. The patient demonstrates cognitive and behavioral deficits that impact the patient's ability to participate in physical therapy. The therapist consults with a neuropsychologist to determine the best strategies for patient management and to optimize interventions and ensure that the best care is provided.*
- A physical therapist consults with another physical therapist.
    - *A physical therapist's examination reveals a vestibular disorder. Although interventions for vestibular disorders fall within the scope of practice of a* physical therapist, *the therapist does not have any experience with vestibular disorders. The patient lives in a rural area and there are no therapists in the area with expertise in the management of patients with vestibular disorders. To ensure that the patient receives optimal care, the physical therapist consults with a physical therapist in another area who is a certified vestibular specialist.*

Comanagement is a common situation in inpatient facilities and with pediatric clients. It occurs when the physical therapist shares responsibility for patient management with providers from other disciplines or with another physical therapist (as in the scenario described above). Comanagement requires collaboration and strong communication due to the shared responsibility for patient care. Examples of comanagement include interdisciplinary care that is provided in an inpatient rehabilitation environment or with school-based therapy services.

When the physical therapist determines that it is appropriate to initiate care, the therapist may directly provide some or all of the interventions or may choose to direct a physical therapist assistant to provide selected interventions. In the event that the physical therapist directs components of the intervention to the physical therapist assistant, the physical therapist remains responsible for all aspects of the physical therapy episode of care and is accountable for the actions of the physical therapist assistant(s).

Prior to initiating interventions, the physical therapist established a plan of care. The plan of care is developed in collaboration with the patient and is based on the examination, evaluation, diagnosis, and prognosis. As indicated in the APTA Defensible Documentation materials, the plan of care includes the following[3]:

- Overall goals stated in functional, measurable terms that indicate the predicted level of improvement in function.
- A statement of interventions/treatments to be provided during the episode of care.
- Duration and frequency of service required to reach the goals.
- Anticipated discharge plans (may be part of the prognosis or written separately).

The physical therapist's plan of care must include succinct, "measurable, functionally driven, and time limited"[1] goals. Goals serve as the tool to which outcomes are compared. This allows for the assessment of the effectiveness of the plan of care and the determination of the patient's progress. A well-written plan of care also delineates the interventions, parameters for each intervention, purpose of the interventions, progression parameters, and, if indicated, precautions.

Intervention

Once the plan of care has been established, direct intervention can begin. As noted earlier, physical therapists may choose to provide the interventions or may direct that interventions be provided by a physical therapist assistant. The *Guide to Physical Therapist Practice* defines interventions as "the purposeful interaction of the physical therapist with an individual—and, when appropriate, with other people involved in the individual's care—to produce changes in the condition that are consistent with the diagnosis and prognosis."[1] Interventions should focus on optimizing the individual's function. Physical therapy interventions fall into the following 9 categories[1]:

- Patient or client instruction (used with every patient and client)
- Airway clearance techniques
- Assistive technology
- Biophysical agents
- Functional training in self-care and domestic, work, community, social, and civic life
- Integumentary repair and protection techniques
- Manual therapy techniques
- Motor function training
- Therapeutic exercise

Outcomes

As physical therapy interventions are initiated, the patient's progress toward the established goals is monitored through the collection of outcomes data. Outcomes data are gathered using tests and observations related to the patient's response to physical therapy interventions. The data (outcomes) are then compared to the initial findings to determine what progress, if any, has occurred. Since outcomes data include a variety of types of data some outcomes data should be noted at every patient encounter. Observations of the patient's functional status, motor control, and more should be made and documented. Other tests are more time consuming and complex and should be scheduled at specific times that correlate with established goals, legal requirements (state practice acts), facility policy, and/or third-party payer mandates. At various times within an episode of care, re-examination may occur to formally document the patient's status and progress, or lack thereof. Based on the findings from the re-examination, the physical therapist may revise the plan of care.

Discharge/Discontinuation of Services

In the plan of care, established as a result of the initial examination and evaluation, the physical therapist will address discharge plans. Depending on several variables (eg, the care setting, the established goals, the patient's progress, the patient's prognosis), the plan may include transfer to another therapy service in another care setting (eg, acute rehab, skilled nursing, outpatient, home health). When established goals are met, discharge from an episode of care occurs. Additionally, discontinuation of physical therapy services may occur without established goals being achieved. When this happens, the physical therapist should document why the established goals were not met.[3] Upon discharge or discontinuation, the patient/client may be given a home exercise program or may be placed on a maintenance therapy program to maintain maximum functional capabilities in the absence of skilled therapeutic intervention. The establishment of a home exercise program, whether during the episode of physical therapy care or at the conclusion of services, should be a part of the plan of care established by the physical therapist.

Physical Therapist and Physical Therapist Assistant Roles

The APTA *Direction and Supervision of the Physical Therapist Assistant*[4] clearly outlines the roles that the physical therapist and physical therapist assistant perform within the Patient/Client Management Model. The physical therapist is the recognized professional who establishes, guides, and directs all aspects of the provision of physical therapy services. It is the responsibility of the physical therapist to interpret referrals; perform the initial examination and evaluation; establish the physical therapy diagnosis, prognosis, and plan of care (including goals and discharge plan); and determine which interventions require the clinical decision-making skill of a physical therapist and which interventions can be provided by a physical therapist assistant. In addition, the physical therapist is responsible for the re-examination of the patient and the revision of the plan of care when indicated. The physical therapist is also directly responsible for ensuring appropriate documentation for all physical therapy services.[4]

As a physical therapist assistant, your role in patient care activities falls within the intervention and outcomes portions of the Patient/Client Management Model. You will implement selected interventions of the plan of care as directed by the physical therapist. You may provide specific interventions from any of the 9 intervention categories listed previously. You must be able to utilize sound clinical reasoning to determine the patient's readiness to engage in the selected interventions and the patient's response(s) to the intervention(s) being providing. You will need to determine when to consult with the physical therapist about the patient's status and progress or lack thereof. Throughout the provision of interventions, you will also need to perform appropriate tests to collect outcomes data to determine the patient's appropriateness to engage in selected interventions and to provide information useful in determining the patient's progress toward the goals established by the physical therapist. As a physical therapist assistant, you will need to modify details of the physical therapist's treatment program to facilitate patient progression within the established plan of care or to ensure the patient's safety and comfort while engaged in the interventions being provided.[5]

Whether interventions are provided by the physical therapist directly or by a physical therapist assistant, the physical therapist remains responsible for all aspects of the physical therapy services. As a physical therapist assistant, you will be responsible for only providing the patient care interventions directed to you by the patient's physical therapist. You will share the responsibility with the physical therapist to ensure that you only provide patient care interventions within your education and skill level and within legal parameters for the state in which you practice.[6-8] It will also be your responsibility to clearly and accurately document all patient care activities that you provide.[4,8]

For the provision of physical therapy services to be efficient and effective, a positive working relationship must exist between the physical therapist and the physical therapist assistant. This type of relationship is characterized by trust and mutual respect, as well as an appreciation for individual differences. A hallmark of a good working relationship is excellent communication.[9,10]

Coordination, Communication, and Documentation

To ensure optimal outcomes from physical therapy services, it is imperative that appropriate coordination of services and communication related to those services occur. Both components can be facilitated through, and should (at a minimum) be outlined in, concise documentation. Collaboration of services includes working with a variety of health care providers and, most importantly, the patient and the patient's family/support structure. Collaboration only occurs in the presence of rich communication. To be able to function within the health care delivery system, you will need to effectively communicate with other members of the health care delivery team. Effective communication includes appropriate verbal and nonverbal communication, as well as accurate documentation. Accurate and effective documentation will provide the foundation upon which all clinical activity occurs. Documentation of the patient's episode of physical therapy care occurs initially with the initial examination/evaluation and throughout the episode of care with interim notes including treatment session notes and re-examination/re-evaluation notes. The final documentation is a discharge summary that provides a summary of the entire episode of care, a description of the patient's status at the time of discharge, and information regarding any additional recommendations for follow-up care (Table 2-2).

Now that we have looked at the Patient/Client Management Model and we have a clear picture of how a patient transitions through an episode of care, let's take a closer look at how documentation plays a part within the provision of physical therapy services.

References

1. American Physical Therapy Association. *Guide to Physical Therapist Practice 3.0.* APTA Website. http://guidetoptpractice.apta.org/content/1/SEC2.body. Updated August 1, 2014. Accessed October 24, 2016.
2. American Physical Therapy Association. *FAQ: direct access at the state level.* APTA Website. http://www.apta.org/StateIssues/DirectAccess/FAQs/. Accessed July 7, 2017.
3. American Physical Therapy Association. *Defensible documentation: components of documentation within the patient/client management model.* APTA Website. http://www.apta.org/Documentation/DefensibleDocumentation/. Accessed January 17, 2017.
4. American Physical Therapy Association. *Guidelines: Physical Therapy Documentation of Patient/Client Management.* BOD G 03-05-16-41. http://www.apta.org/uploadedFiles/APTAorg/About_Us/Policies/Practice/DocumentationPatientClientManagement.pdf. Updated December 14, 2009. Accessed July 7, 2017.
5. American Physical Therapy Association. *Direction and supervision of the physical therapist assistant.* HOD P06-05-18-26. http://www.apta.org/uploadedFiles/APTAorg/Practice_and_Patient_Care/Movement_System/MovementSystemSummit_Prereadings.pdf Accessed July 7, 2017.
6. American Physical Therapy Association. *A Normative Model of Physical Therapist Assistant Education.* Alexandria, VA: American Physical Therapy Association; 2007.
7. American Physical Therapy Association. *Minimum required skills of physical therapist assistant graduates at entry-level.* BOD G11-08-09-18. https://www.apta.org/uploadedFiles/APTAorg/About_Us/Policies/BOD/Education/MinReqSkillsPTGrad.pdf. Accessed January 14, 2017.
8. American Physical Therapy Association. *Standards of ethical conduct for the physical therapist assistant.* APTA Website. https://www.apta.org/uploadedFiles/APTAorg/About_Us/Policies/Ethics/CodeofEthics.pdf. Accessed January 14, 2017.
9. Holcomb S. *Recipe for effective teamwork: why some PT/ PTA pairings thrive, to patient's ultimate benefit.* PT Magazine. February 2009. http://www.apta.org/PTinMotion/2009/2/. Accessed January 15, 2017.
10. American Physical Therapy Association. *PT/PTA teamwork: models in delivering patient care.* APTA Website. http://www.apta.org/SupervisionTeamwork/Models/. Accessed January 15, 2017.

Table 2-2

Episode of Care Documentation

Documentation Notes	Written By	When	Includes	Purpose
Initial	Physical therapist	At the initiation of an episode of care prior to provision of any interventions	• A description of the patient status • Findings from the examination • The physical therapist's evaluation • The physical therapist's plan of care	Provides data needed for the physical therapist to determine the plan of care
Interim—Treatment Session	Physical therapist or physical therapist assistant who provided the interventions	At every patient care encounter		
Interim—Re-examination/Re-evaluation	Physical therapist			
Discharge Summary	Physical therapist	At the end of an episode of care		

Review Questions

1. Create a concept map that depicts an episode of physical therapy care from the point of entry through discharge.

2. Describe how patients access physical therapy care. Provide 3 examples of how a patient might gain access to a physical therapist.

3. Define and describe the 5 elements of the Patient/Client Management Model.

4. Next to each component of the Patient/Client Management Model, indicate whether the physical therapist (indicate with PT), the physical therapist assistant (indicate with PTA), or both participate(s) in that process.
   __________ Examination
   __________ Evaluation
   __________ Diagnosis
   __________ Prognosis
   __________ Intervention
   __________ Outcomes

5. Describe the types of decisions made by the physical therapist during the evaluation process.

6. List the essential components of a plan of care.

7. What is the importance of outcomes measures in patient/client management?

8. Describe the role of the physical therapist assistant in the physical therapy process. List the responsibilities of the physical therapist assistant within that role.

Application Exercises

I. Reference the physical therapy practice act for your state of residence for language regarding direct access. Are there any restrictions or provisions related to direct access in the practice act? If so, what are they?

II. Reference the physical therapy practice act for your state or residence for language regarding documentation. What are the responsibilities of the physical therapist assistant regarding documentation? What, if any, are the restrictions placed upon the physical therapist assistant regarding documentation? Compare your state practice act with a practice act from a different state. What are the similarities? What are the differences? Discuss how these differing requirements can impact the operation of physical therapy in a variety of settings.

III. Interview a friend or family member who has received physical therapy services. Ask him or her to describe how he or she entered the physical therapy care system. Ask him or her to describe the process as he or she remembers it. Compare the information that you receive with the experiences reported by other interviews performed by your classmates.

Chapter 3

Reasons for Documenting

Mia L. Erickson, PT, EdD, CHT, ATC

KEY TERMS Maintenance therapy | Medicaid | Medicare | Objective data | Reasonable and necessary criteria | Reimbursement | Skilled care (services) | Subjective data

Chapter Objectives

After reading this chapter, the reader will be able to do the following:

1. List the major reasons for documenting.
2. Identify the types of patient data found in a medical record.
3. Explain how clinical decision making can be articulated in a medical record.
4. Explain the role of the physical therapist assistant in the clinical decision-making process.
5. Describe the reasonable and necessary criteria.
6. Differentiate between skilled care and maintenance therapy.
7. Explain how to document the patient's response to treatment.

Imagine that you are working as a physical therapist assistant in a small outpatient clinic. For the last 6 weeks, you and your supervising physical therapist have been working with a 35-year-old man who was recently involved in a motor vehicle accident. He sustained a concussion and multiple fractures including the left femur and radius. Initially, he was unable to bear weight through either extremity and required a wheelchair as his primary mode of mobility. He had significant loss in range of motion and was unable to perform self-care, home/community mobility, and work activities. He has been making excellent progress and is now able to walk using one crutch and has resumed most of his normal activities of daily living. The physical therapist with whom you are working receives a call from the patient's insurance company stating that they are going to deny payment for physical therapy services. To have additional therapy services approved, the clinic must submit adequate documentation showing that further skilled services are medically necessary.

Legal and Ethical Responsibility

As a physical therapist assistant, documentation will be one of the most important things you do. In health care, documentation provides a legal record of care, facilitates communication among health care providers, and serves as a source of information for clinical research.[1] Both state and federal laws mandate recording health care provided to an individual. Facilities and organizations providing com-

Erickson ML, McKnight R. *Documentation Basics for the Physical Therapist Assistant, Third Edition* (pp. 19-28)

ponents of the Patient/Client Management Model discussed in Chapter 2 have policies pertaining to documentation.

Medical records are legal documents, and any entry you make into the medical record becomes part of that legal document; therefore, it is important that your documentation is accurate, legible, and completely depicts the patient's condition and intervention provided. Be aware that a patient's medical records can be subpoenaed and used as evidence in a variety of legal matters. These include motor vehicle accidents, workers' compensation or disability claims, and malpractice suits brought against you or other health care providers. In malpractice lawsuits, documentation is the clinician's first line of defense. Good documentation can stop a lawsuit in its tracks, and poor documentation can be "powerful evidence in support of a suit, even when the accusations are frivolous."[2] Consider the following as a rule of thumb: "If it isn't documented, it didn't happen."

In addition to legal obligations, maintaining accurate, timely, well-written patient records is considered one of your ethical duties as a physical therapist assistant. The *Standards of Ethical Conduct for the Physical Therapist Assistant* states, "Physical therapist assistants shall ensure that documentation for their interventions accurately reflects the nature and extent of the services provided."[3]

Reimbursement

Reimbursement means "to pay back" for a service that has been provided.[4] In health care, either the patient or a third party (eg, an insurance company, government agency such as Medicare) pays for services. Medicare and Medicaid began requiring documentation for reimbursement in physical therapy in the 1960s.[1] Soon after that, Medicare began a restructuring process and started requiring rehabilitation facilities to not only maintain documentation, but also to submit the records for review by Medicare auditors. The purpose of these reviews was to determine whether physical therapy services provided to Medicare beneficiaries met requirements for reimbursement. As the US health care delivery system has evolved over the last decades, third-party reimbursement from all payers has become another reason for documenting patient care. Reimbursement from third-party payers can be dependent upon documentation in that, to receive payment, the documentation must support the services provided. Consider the patient case discussed earlier in this chapter. Continuation of his physical therapy benefits is based largely on how well the clinicians have documented his improvement and the need for ongoing services. Communication with third-party payers through appropriate documentation has been called the "key to securing reimbursement."[5]

Record Patient Data

One of the primary reasons for documenting physical therapy services is to maintain a record of patient data. These data should reflect the entire episode of patient care, from start to finish, beginning with an initial examination performed by the physical therapist and ending with a discharge summary. During the initial examination, the physical therapist collects and records data pertaining to the patient's current condition. These include both subjective and objective information. The history-taking portion of the initial examination provides the physical therapist with subjective information. It includes what the patient, family member, or caregiver says pertaining to the patient's condition. History of the current condition, mechanism of injury, date of onset, and history of a similar problem are all examples of subjective information gathered during the initial examination. Other subjective information collected at this point should include a thorough medical history, a review of the patient's living situation, chief complaints (including his or her activity limitations and restrictions in his or her ability to participate in normal life roles or tasks), and his or her goals for physical therapy. Information related to the patient's functional status can be gleaned through direct questioning by the physical therapist or through the use of patient self-report measures. Self-report measures are questionnaires that ask the patient to rate his or her ability to perform functional tasks. Data from these questionnaires provide the physical therapist and physical therapist assistant with information about patient functioning from the patient's perspective.

In addition to subjective information, documented data should include objective information or results from the systems review and objective tests and measurements. Examples of these types of objective data include measurements of range of motion, strength, sensation, girth, balance, and functional status (eg, walking, transferring, performing activities such as self-care and home management). While data from self-report measures of function are often considered part of the subjective information, data from observable patient performance of a functional task are considered objective information. Objective data provide additional information to help identify and measure the extent of the patient's impairments, activity limitations, and participation restrictions. Self-report measures, observation of functional performance, and performance-based measures can be used together to provide information about the patient's functional status.

A record of the patient's functional status provides particularly valuable information regarding the effects of the disease or injury on the patient's normal activities and lifestyle. Furthermore, individuals reviewing medical records deem the patient's functional status as being more meaningful than documentation of impairments alone.

Although impairment data are necessary, documenting function, including activity limitations and participation restrictions, provides reviewers with specific contextual information regarding the impact of injury on the patient's lifestyle.

Both subjective and objective data provide physical therapists and physical therapist assistants with baseline measurements with which future measurements can be compared.[6] Information taken from the patient, as well as objective measurements, are not only documented during the initial examination, but also during subsequent physical therapy sessions. In subsequent sessions, data are recorded in the form of treatment or interim notes, progress reports, or, in the case of discharge from physical therapy services, a discharge summary. In any event, any data collected after the initial examination should be recorded. It will be compared with that found in the initial examination. These comparisons allow the medical record to reflect both subjective (patient comments) and objective (data from tests/measurements) changes in the patient's status.

Records of patient data are important to others involved in the patient's care. Health care providers such as physicians, nurses, occupational and speech therapists, and case managers, among others, are often interested in a patient's status and therefore might examine physical therapy documentation. Physicians might be interested in how far a patient can walk prior to deciding on discharge from the hospital. Nurses might be interested in a patient's ability to transfer out of the bed, whereas case managers might want to examine equipment needs or return-to-work status; therefore, documentation serves as a useful tool for facilitating communication across disciplines. In addition to other health care providers, third-party payers are interested in records of patient data.

Accurate records of patient data also aid in our ability to analyze and study patient outcomes. Outcomes are defined as the end result of patient/client management.[7] Collection of outcomes data is an important area of physical therapy practice, and it is necessary to support and validate the physical therapy services provided. Outcomes data are also necessary to support evidence-based practice. For example, analysis of patient outcomes can allow us to determine the effectiveness of physical therapy interventions. Use of standard terms, such as those provided by the *International Classification of Functioning, Disability and Health* in our data collection can also support outcomes data collection.[8]

Record Patient Care

Your documentation will also serve as a record of the care you provided to your patients. Interventions are divided into 3 categories. The first is procedural interventions. These are considered direct interventions and include those related to direct patient care, such as modalities, physical agents (eg, ice, heat), massage, stretching exercises, strengthening exercises, gait training, and transfer training. The second category is coordination and communication. This is more indirect but is still an important aspect of patient care. Examples include communicating with family members, other health care providers, or any other individual involved in the care of the patient. Phone calls, relevant conversations regarding the patient, and collaboration with other providers, including the physical therapist, must also be documented as part of the patient's record. The third category is patient/client-related instruction. This category includes teaching that was provided to the patient, family, or caregiver as well as his or her understanding or response to the teaching. Both physical therapists and physical therapist assistants are responsible for accurately recording services provided in each of these 3 categories.

Documented interventions serve to support treatment that was billed for a given date of service. Third-party payers may perform a documentation audit to assure that the treatment provided and billed is supported by the clinician's documentation. Inaccurate or incomplete documentation that does not support daily charges may be construed as fraud or abuse and must be avoided.

Accurately recording patient care is also necessary where electronic billing and documentation software are integrated. In these situations, the patient's charges are generated based on the interventions that the therapist provided and documented in the day's note. Incomplete or inaccurate documentation may generate too many or too few charges to the patient's account. Additionally, a patient may be charged for a service not provided. Again, these inconsistencies can prompt an audit, which can result in fines, repayment, or accusations of abuse or fraud, so it is very important that the record accurately reflects all aspects of the care provided to the patient.

Another reason for documenting patient care is to keep a record for other therapists in the event of your absence. In the event of an emergency where a physical therapy provider is unable to come to work, another physical therapist or physical therapist assistant should be able to pick up the record and provide the appropriate patient care. This maintains consistency of care across providers.

In addition to specific patient care provided, it is important to document the patient's response to treatment. This can be done in a variety of ways. Thinking in terms of disablement, response to treatment should provide information as to how the interventions are positively or negatively influencing the patient's impairments, activity limitations, or participation restrictions. For example, a physical therapist could record the following:

Dynamic balance training and lower-extremity strengthening exercises have allowed the patient to improve balance as measured by the Berg Balance Scale and the patient is now at less risk for falls.

In this example, the physical therapist documented the patient's overall response to treatment in terms of impairments (improved balance) and function (less risk of falls). Consider the following example written by a physical therapist assistant:

Upon arrival, the patient was complaining of 6/10 pain in the right buttock and leg and was having difficulty sitting. Following modalities and extension exercises, the pain decreased to 3/10 and was no longer radiating down the patient's leg.

When the response to treatment is documented in this manner, the note reflects how the interventions brought about a change in the patient's status, and it supports treatment effectiveness. Being specific in the patient's response can show a third-party payer how the patient is improving and how the treatment is influencing impairments and function.

Documenting response to treatment can serve as a record of unexpected events that may have taken place and your response. For example, when a patient returns for a therapy visit and has increased soreness after performing his home exercise program, the physical therapist assistant can make adjustments within the plan of care to lower the exercise intensity. Patient complaints should be documented, and the therapist's actions in response to the patient's complaints should also be documented. The therapist's response to an adverse event may not always be directed toward the patient. Consider the following example:

A physical therapist goes to see a patient 4 weeks post total knee arthroplasty for a re-evaluation in the patient's home. The patient is complaining of severe knee pain, swelling, nausea, redness, elevated skin temperature, and white drainage from the incision. Upon observation, the physical therapist believes that the patient has an infection and calls the physician.

The physical therapist should document the events that took place, the observations, any assessments, and his or her action. Documenting response to treatment and your actions, when appropriate, helps to show patient management and clinical decision making in response to positive or negative events.

Provide Proof That Care Is Reasonable and Necessary

Our documentation must provide evidence that physical therapy services are reasonable and necessary. The Centers for Medicare & Medicaid Services has set forth the following criteria that need to be met for services to be considered reasonable and necessary[9]:

- "The services shall be considered under accepted standards of medical practice to be a specific and effective treatment for the patient's condition."
- "The services shall be of such a level of complexity and sophistication or the condition of the patient shall be such that the services required can be safely and effectively performed only by a therapist, or in the case of physical therapy and occupational therapy by or under the supervision of a therapist."
- "While a beneficiary's particular medical condition is a valid factor in deciding if skilled therapy services are needed, a beneficiary's diagnosis or prognosis cannot be the sole factor in deciding that a service is or is not skilled. The key issue is whether the skills of a therapist are needed to treated the illness or injury, or whether the services can be carried out by nonskilled personnel."
- "The amount, frequency, and duration of the services must be reasonable under accepted standards of practice. The contractor shall consult local professionals or the state or national therapy associations in the development of any utilization guidelines."

Documentation to justify reasonable and necessary services includes initial documentation that describes the patient's pathology, impairments, activity limitations, and participation restrictions. The documentation includes a description of how the impairments have led to limitations in a patient's activity level or restrictions in a patient's ability to participate in normal life roles or tasks. Documentation outlines a specific plan of care or interventions aimed at addressing these limitations, and it includes ongoing reassessments to show changes in status. The documentation must convey how the interventions are influencing the patient's condition. Furthermore, the documentation must show how the interventions provided required the unique and complex skills or decision making of a therapist. Finally, the frequency and duration of services should be consistent with what would be considered appropriate for the case.

In most cases, the physical therapist provides evidence that services are reasonable and necessary in the initial documentation. The physical therapist assistant, however, plays an important role in recognizing when the intervention is no longer reasonable and necessary. For example, intervention may no longer be reasonable and necessary if any of the following occurs: (1) the patient has met all of the goals that have been established by the physical therapist; (2) the patient is no longer benefiting from the intervention; or (3) the services can be carried out through home exercise instructions or by untrained personnel. Treatment might also exceed the reasonable and necessary criteria if a patient, family member, or caregiver has unrealistic expectations for recovery.[10] Documentation showing objective, comparative data can help to provide evidence that a patient is progressing toward the goals stated in the plan of care. Documentation can then further support the need for subsequent or continued interventions under the reasonable and necessary criteria, or it can provide justification for discontinuing physical therapy services.

Provide Proof of Skilled Care

Medicare has provided definitions for skilled care and documentation criteria.[11] When determining if a service is skilled, it is always important to first consider the service being provided and whether it reaches a level of complexity that it must be carried out by a therapist or under the supervision of a therapist for both safety and effectiveness. As stated in the previous section, the patient's medical condition is a valid factor in determining if skilled services are needed; however, it is never the only factor.

There may be times when an unskilled service could be considered a skilled service. This is the case when a patient's medical condition, comorbidities, or complicating factors are such that the service should be provided or supervised by a therapist for safety and effectiveness. Consider passive exercises for example. In some cases, passive exercise would be considered unskilled; however, if a patient presents with a humeral fracture and requires passive elbow exercises, then, due to the condition, the intervention would be considered skilled. Unskilled services are often known as maintenance therapy. Maintenance therapy services can be provided by a nonlicensed individual, such as a family member or caregiver who has had some training from a skilled professional, or by the patient through independent home exercises. Medicare and other third-party payers do not reimburse for maintenance services.[12]

Documentation in all cases must be thorough enough to show a reviewer that the services were skilled. The *Medicare Benefit Policy Manual* outlined documentation requirements to support skilled care determinations.[11] According to these guidelines, there should be sufficient documentation to help a reviewer determine the following: (1) the service requires the skills of a therapist to be considered safe and effective; (2) the service is reasonable and necessary and consistent with the nature and severity of the illness or injury, the patient's medical needs, and accepted standards of practice; and (3) the service is appropriate in terms of duration and quantity and is designed to meet a documented therapeutic goal. In addition, the medical record should provide thorough documentation of the history and physical examination pertinent to the patient's care (including response to treatment from previously administered skilled interventions), the skilled services provided to the patient, the response to the skilled services provided during the current visit, the plan for future care based on the rationale of prior results, a rationale that explains the need for skilled service in light of the condition, the complexity of the services provided, and any other pertinent patient characteristics that would support the need for skilled services.[11]

These documentation requirements state that the patient's record should be accurate and specific in documenting the patient's response to skilled care, avoiding vague and subjective descriptions such as "tolerated treatment well," and "continue with plan of care" since these phrases do not adequately describe the patient's response in objective terms.[11] Rather, requirements state that objective measurements of physical outcomes and/or a clear description of the patient's response(s) that occurs as a result of the skilled service should be provided. This allows for all concerned to be able to follow the results of the skilled services provided.[11]

Demonstrate the Clinical Decision-Making Process

From initial examination to discharge, physical therapy documentation should provide a picture of the clinician's decision-making processes and clinical judgment.[2,10,12] Documentation that demonstrates clinical decision making also improves the provider's credibility with third-party payers.[5] An individual who does not know the patient should be able to read the physical therapy records and identify a logical, stepwise progression from initial examination to discharge. Lewis[2] indicated, "documentation of all elements of the Patient/Client Management Model... should harmonize." Documentation should reflect logical decisions and sound judgment by showing direct links between subjective remarks; objective measures of impairments activity limitation and participation restriction; therapy goals; skilled interventions; responses to the skilled interventions in objective, measurable terms; changes in interventions, when appropriate; and a rationale for discharge.

Both the physical therapist and physical therapist assistant have specific roles in making sure that this occurs, as follows:

- Data collected during the initial examination should be reflected in the plan of care. For example, goals written by the physical therapist should reflect impairments (ie, decreased range of motion, decreased strength), activity limitations (ie, difficulty transferring, decreased independence with gait), and participation restrictions (ie, unable to work) identified during the initial examination (physical therapist role).
- The plan of care should include physical therapy interventions that are aimed at reducing the identified impairments, activity limitations, and participation restrictions (physical therapist role).
- Changes in patient status should prompt changes in the plan of care (physical therapist and physical therapist assistant role to recognize and record changes in patient status, physical therapist assistant role to communicate changes to the physical therapist, and physical therapist role to adjust the plan of care based on patient changes).

The physical therapist assistant can further contribute to the decision-making process by collecting pertinent subjective and objective patient data in visits following the initial examination, before and after providing interventions. Subjective data often gathered and recorded by a physical therapist assistant include the following:

- Asking the patient about his or her response to a previous treatment.
- Inquiring about compliance with a home exercise program.
- Asking the patient whether the treatment has improved his or her function.

When asking a patient whether the treatment has improved his or her function, it is important to refer back to the initial documentation to see what limitations the patient had when he or she started the episode of care. That way, additional inquiries can be directed at specific activity limitations and participation restrictions.

Prior to collecting objective data through tests and measurements, it is important to see what measurements were taken during the initial evaluation. These initial measurements serve as a baseline for determining future measurements that are needed and for which future measurements should be compared. In addition, it is important to try to speak with the physical therapist about the patient prior to the treatment session. At that time, one should ask whether additional tests and measurements are needed. Objective data often gathered by a physical therapist assistant include but are not limited to the following:

- Goniometric measurements
- Manual muscle testing
- Functional status (bed mobility, transfers, gait)

The physical therapist assistant records subjective patient comments and results of relevant tests and measurements in interim notes or daily notes. These notes help to tell the story of the patient and can lend support to patient improvement. Subjective and objective findings that warrant a re-evaluation, changes in the plan of care, or discharge should also be provided in the documentation by the physical therapist assistant and communicated to the physical therapist.

When there is consistency between the initial examination and subsequent notes, the clinical decision-making process is more apparent. Ongoing documentation of subjective remarks and objective findings tells the story of the patient's response to therapy. In addition, consistency between initial and subsequent documentation makes it easier for the clinician(s) to identify progress or lack thereof. This also allows the physical therapist to easily update goals and interventions as needed.

References

1. Inaba M, Jones SL. Medical documentation for third-party payers. *Phys Ther.* 1977;57(7):791-794.
2. Lewis DK. Do the write thing: document everything. *PT Magazine.* 2002;10(7):30-34.
3. American Physical Therapy Association House of Delegates. *Standards of Ethical Conduct for the Physical Therapist Assistant.* HOD S06-09-20-18 [Amended HOD S06-00-13-24; HOD 06-91-06-07; Initial HOD 06-82-04-08] [Standard]. APTA Website. http://www.apta.org/uploadedFiles/APTAorg/About_Us/Policies/Ethics/StandardsEthicalConductPTA.pdf. Accessed July 8, 2017.
4. *Definition of reimbursement.* Dictionary.com Website. http://www.dictionary.com/browse/reimbursement. Accessed July 8, 2017.
5. Baeten AM. Documentation: the reviewer perspective. *Top Geriatr Rehabil.* 1997;13(1):14-22.
6. Hebert LA. Basics of Medicare documentation for physical therapy. *Clinical Management in Physical Therapy.* 1981;1(3):13-14.
7. American Physical Therapy Association. *Guide to Physical Therapist Practice 3.0.* APTA Website. http://guidetoptpractice.apta.org/content/1/SEC2.body. Updated August 1, 2014. Accessed October 24, 2016.
8. Goode N. The reliable resource: physical therapy documentation. *PT Magazine.* 1999;7(9):30-31.
9. Centers for Medicare & Medicaid Services. *Medicare Benefit Policy Manual. Chapter 15-Covered Medical and Other Health Services.* CMS.gov website. https://www.cms.gov/Regulations-and-Guidance/Guidance/Manuals/Downloads/bp102c15.pdf. Updated July 11, 2017. Accessed July 8, 2017.
10. Redgate N, Foto M. Pay by the rules: avoid Medicare audits and reduce payment denials with a sound strategy and proper documentation. *Physical Therapy Products.* 2003;October/November:28-30.
11. Centers for Medicare & Medicaid Services. *Medicare Benefit Policy Manual. Chapter 8-Coverage of Extended Care (SNF) Services Under Hospital Insurance.* CMS.gov website. https://www.cms.gov/Regulations-and-Guidance/Guidance/Manuals/downloads/bp102c08.pdf. Updated October 13, 2016. Accessed July 8, 2017.
12. Moorhead JF, Clifford J. Determining medical necessity of outpatient physical therapy services. *Am J Med Qual.* 1992;7(3):81-84.

Review Questions

1. List reasons for documenting.

2. Review the *Standards of Ethical Conduct for the Physical Therapist Assistant* (http://www.apta.org/uploadedFiles/APTAorg/About_Us/Policies/Ethics/StandardsEthicalConductPTA.pdf) and identify your professional obligation(s) that pertain to documentation.

3. What are some examples of subjective and objective data that can be gathered by a physical therapist assistant?

4. How can a clinician integrate the clinical decision-making process in his or her documentation?

5. Provide some examples of how a physical therapist assistant can assist in showing clinical decision making in the medical record.

6. What are the criteria for determining whether a treatment or intervention is reasonable and necessary?

7. List some examples of how a physical therapist or physical therapist assistant should document a patient's response to treatment.

8. What is the difference between skilled care and maintenance therapy? Provide an example of each.

9. What is the role of the physical therapist assistant in determining medical necessity?

10. How does the patient's rehabilitation potential influence his or her need for medically necessary skilled care?

Application Exercises

Read through the following initial examination/evaluation performed and documented by the physical therapist, and answer the questions that follow.

Date: March 15, 2017

Patient: David White

Pr: 27 y.o. s/p (L) wrist and ankle fx; Referral: Begin gentle wrist and ankle AROM and PROM; May begin using crutches with platform for (L) UE. PWB 50% on (L) LE.

S: *HPI*: 4 weeks s/p fall (~25') from a logging truck landing on his (L) side (2/1/17). Pt. sustained fx of the (L) distal radius and ulna and (L) distal tibia and fibula. Pt. underwent ORIF for the wrist and ankle immediately after the injury. He was placed in a short-arm cast for the UE and short-leg cast for the LE. He was NWB on the (L) LE initially and has been unable to use crutches due to not being allowed to bear weight on the affected UE. He was hospitalized for 5 days following the injury. While hospitalized, he received PT to learn how to negotiate his w/c and perform transfers. Both casts were removed yesterday and his ankle was placed in a removable splint. He reports taking ibuprofen PRN for pain.

C/C: Pain and stiffness in (L) UE and LE with decreased functional use of both. Doesn't like using w/c for mobility. Unable to work. Requiring assist with self-care activities and home management.

Living situation: Right-hand dominant; Lives with wife and 2 small children in single-level home with 2 steps @ entrance and hand rail on the (R). Pt. is unable to drive and is relying on his wife and mother for transportation.

Work history: Prior to injury, pt. was employed as a construction worker. He has been off work since the injury.

PMH/family history: Pt. reports being in good general health. Prior to injury pt. was independent in all functional activities in and around the home. No significant PMH or history of fracture. Family history is (+) for OA.

Social/health habits: Reports being a nonsmoker and nondrinker.

Self-report of function: DASH score: 85%; FAAM score: 9%;

Global rating of function: 9%.

Pt.'s goals: Return to previous level of function and RTW ASAP. Learn to ambulate with crutches.

O: Systems Review: *Cardiovascular system*: HR: 80 bpm, RR: 12, BP 125/75;

Integumentary system: Healed scars on the volar surface of the (L) wrist and lateral surface of the (L) lower leg. Scars are pink, slightly raised (<2mm), and slightly adhered to the underlying tissue.

Neuromuscular system: Impaired, see below;

Musculoskeletal system: Impaired, see below.

Communication and cognition: No impairments identified, able to communicate without difficulty.

Tests and Measures:

		AROM	PROM
(L) wrist:	Flexion	0°	25°
	Extension	10°	15°
	UD	10°	15°
	RD	15°	15°
	Supination	30°	35°
	Pronation	40°	45°
(L) hand:	Patient can perform a full fist but it is difficult due to edema. Thumb IP, MCP, and CMC AROM is WNL		
(L) knee:		0-100°	0-110°
(L) ankle:	DF	-10°	-5°
	PF	20°	25°
	Inversion	5°	5°
	Eversion	0°	5°

AROM: (R) UE and LE WNL; (L) shoulder, elbow, and hip WNL.

Strength: (R) UE and LE 5/5; grip strength (#2 handle setting) 110#; (L) shoulder and hip 4/5; (L) elbow, wrist, knee, and ankle deferred 2° to acuity.

Girth: wrist figure 8 (R): 36 cm (L): 37.2 cm; ankle figure 8 (R): 42 cm (L): 44.1 cm.

Sensation: Diminished light touch at the (L) wrist and ankle incisions

Circulation: 2+ at radial and dorsal pedal arteries on the (L).

Special Tests: N/A @ this time 2° to acuity.

Gait: Ambulates 50' PWB 50% (L) LE using crutches with (L) UE platform using step to gait pattern with CGAx1 for sequencing and balance.

Transfers: (I) bed to and from chair, chair to and from toilet, sit to and from stand; all PWB on (L) LE.

Bed Mobility: (I) all areas.

Tx and HEP: Ther Ex x 30 minutes including AROM and PROM for (L) wrist for flexion, extension, pronation, and supination and for (L) ankle DF and PF, used opposite foot for self PROM of ankle; performed AROM for all digits and thumb; initiated compression glove for edema to be worn at night; instructed pt. in elevation and compression wrapping for ankle and wrist; Gait training x 15 minutes including instruction in use of crutches. Pt. performed all ex. x 20 reps (I) and verbalized understanding of all precautions.

A: 27 y.o. RHD male 4 wks s/p fall where he sustained fx to the (L) wrist and ankle. Now decreased AROM, PROM, strength, and weightbearing restrictions are causing inability to ambulate, perform self-care, drive, or perform home management tasks without assistance. He is also unable to work @ this time. Pt. demonstrates excellent motivation and good potential for full recovery. No comorbidities identified that could affect outcome at this time.

Problem List:

1. Decreased AROM and PROM of the (L) hand, wrist, forearm, knee, and ankle
2. Edema in the (L) hand and ankle limiting ROM
3. Decreased strength in the (L) UE and LE
4. Limited (I) in mobility including ambulation
5. Unable to ascend and descend stairs
6. Decreased (I) with self-care
7. Decreased (I) with home management
8. Unable to drive
9. Unable to work

Anticipated Goals and Expected Outcomes:

At the end of 4 weeks, pt. will:

1. Increase AROM 20-25° for the wrist, forearm, knee, and ankle to improve use of UE and LE during functional activities.
2. Decrease edema by 0.5 cm for the wrist and ankle to improve ROM.
3. Perform a full fist without limitations.
4. Ambulate 200' with crutches with (L) UE platform PWB 50% on (L) LE independently.
5. Ascend and descend stairs with supervision and assistive device.
6. Perform all self-care independently.
7. Improve his score on the FAAM 8-16%.
8. Improve his DASH score 15%.

At the end of 16 weeks (time of d/c), pt. will:

1. Achieve the following AROM: wrist extension 70°, wrist flexion 80°, supination 75°, pronation 75°, knee 0-150°, ankle DF 10°, and ankle PF 50° to allow use during basic care, home tasks, and work activities.
2. Increase strength in the (L) wrist, knee, and ankle to 4/5 to allow normal function for RTW.
3. Achieve grip strength to 80% of (R) to allow use during basic care, home tasks, and work activities.
4. Ambulate independently on all surfaces without an assistive device.
5. Ascend and descend a flight of stairs independently without an assistive device.
6. Demonstrate (I) self-care.
7. Demonstrate (I) in home management tasks.
8. Drive without restrictions.
9. RTW @ previous level of employment.

P: See pt. 3x/wk for next 3-4 mos. to provide skilled services including instruction in safe, appropriate therapeutic exercise program and progression, use of assistive device and gait training as ordered, retraining in functional mobility to prepare for return to normal lifestyle and RTW. Will progress pt. as tolerated when appropriate and according to MD orders. Pt. is in agreement with the above stated plan.

John Smith, PT

1. List 5 of the patient's impairments.
2. List 2 of the patient's activity limitations and 2 of his participation restrictions.
3. In this example, how are the patient's impairments creating activity limitations and participation restriction?
4. List 5 pieces of subjective data found in the examination.
5. List 5 pieces of objective data found in the examination.
6. What other providers/individuals might be interested in looking at this patient's note(s)?
7. What interventions were provided to the patient on this initial date of service?
8. How did the physical therapist describe the need for skilled care?
9. What information would you need to provide in a progress note for this patient to show medical necessity and the need for further skilled care?
10. What examples can you see in this note that help in supporting the clinical decision-making process used by this physical therapist?

Chapter 4

Documentation Formats

Mia L. Erickson, PT, EdD, CHT, ATC

KEY TERMS Assessment | Functional outcome report | Individualized Education Plan | Individualized Family Service Plan | Individuals with Disabilities in Education Act | Narrative | Objective | Plan | Problem-oriented medical record | SOAP note | Subjective

KEY ABBREVIATIONS A | FOR | IDEA | IEP | IFSP | O | P | POMR | S | SOAP

Chapter Objectives

After reading this chapter, the reader will be able to do the following:

1. Describe each documentation format.
2. Examine the different physical therapy documentation formats.
3. Explain the advantages and disadvantages of different documentation formats.
4. Differentiate between information found in the S (subjective), O (objective), A (assessment), and P (plan) portions of a SOAP note.
5. Identify the positive and negative aspects of using forms and templates.
6. Recognize the need for adapting clinical documentation into a given format.

Documentation in physical therapy practice can take on a variety of formats depending on the type of patients being treated, practice setting, type of facility, state laws and practice acts, reimbursement requirements, and electronic medical record system being used. Historically, there have been several formats used in physical therapy practice, such as narrative reports, the problem-oriented medical record, the SOAP note, and the functional outcomes report (FOR; Figure 4-1). While a brief discussion of each will be provided, it is important to point out that, as the health care system transitions to electronic medical record keeping, one will have to be flexible in adapting to the templates provided by the software available at the site; therefore, it is important for new clinicians to have an overview of basic formats so that they can be able to adapt to a given computer interface.

Narrative

In narrative documentation, the clinician describes the patient encounter in paragraph format.

Narrative Example #1

Date: 03/30/17

Patient: David White

Pt. RTC reporting no adverse effects from treatment last visit or from HEP. He stated that he feels as though his wrist and ankle are moving better and the edema in the hand has decreased. He reports improvement in his gait, ability to shower (I) using a plastic chair in the tub, and ability to

Erickson ML, McKnight R. *Documentation Basics for the Physical Therapist Assistant, Third Edition* (pp. 29-40)

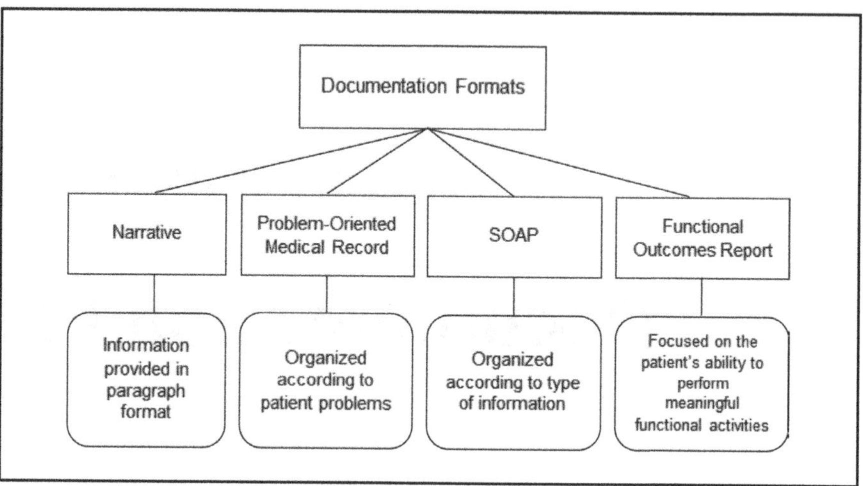

Figure 4-1. Documentation formats.

dress himself. AROM of the (L) wrist is as follows: flexion 30°, extension 30°, UD 15°, RD 20°, supination 45°, and pronation 60°; (L) knee: 0-135°; (L) ankle: DF 0°, PF 45°. Figure 8 wrist girth is 35.5 cm and ankle figure 8 girth is 43 cm on the (L). Pt. ambulated 1000' (I) with crutches using (L) UE platform, PWB 50% on the (L) LE. Tx consisted of gentle AROM and PROM for 30' to the (L) wrist and forearm in the directions of flexion, extension, supination, and pronation and to the (L) ankle for DF, PF, inversion, and eversion. Pt. also performed AROM for the fingers to improve the ability to make a tight fist. Pt. has made improvements in AROM and has decreased edema. His functional activity has also improved per subjective report. Will continue to have pt. perform his HEP and RTC on 4/5/17.

Bill Jones, PTA

Several problems with the narrative record have been reported. First, narrative notes can lack structure, making the writer prone to omit important details. In addition, there is a high degree of note-writing variability among clinicians.[1] When medical notes lack structure and vary between clinicians, it becomes very difficult for others to read and locate necessary information. For example, it would be very time consuming for a physician or case manager to sort through a chart filled with unstructured narrative entries to locate information regarding the patient's ability to transfer or ambulate. Furthermore, following the clinician's problem-solving process can be difficult in narrative reports.[2] Nevertheless, the use of narrative notes still occurs, and ways to improve readability with this format have been suggested. First, when using the narrative format, Quinn and Gordon[1] recommended developing an outline of information to cover so that important details are not omitted. Also, using headings and subheadings can make information easier to find. Whether to use headings and which headings to use can often be left to the discretion of the individual clinician, but some facilities may have policies as to which headings should and should not be used.

There are times when the narrative format is the most appropriate format to use. These include describing a sequence of events, brief interactions with patients, conversations with other health care providers, or any other situation that requires a detailed explanation and no other documentation formats are appropriate (see Narrative Example #2). These are also useful when documenting a cancellation, refusal to participate, or missed visit. In these instances, you can simply describe the situation and how it affects the patient in a brief paragraph or narrative note. Narrative notes are sometimes the easiest to use when you just need to describe the details of a situation and you are trying to paint a vivid description of what happened. The narrative format can be used in both paper and electronic medical records.

Narrative Example #2

Date: 04/01/17

Patient: David White

Spoke with patient's physician today regarding the amount of weight bearing that he is allowed to perform when ambulating with the platform crutches. The physician stated that his fracture sites on the radius and ulna are stable and healing well, and he can perform weight bearing as tolerated on the UE. Will have patient continue to use crutches with platform on the (L), allowing him to bear weight through the UE as instructed by the physician.

John Smith, PT

Problem-Oriented Medical Record

The POMR was introduced by Lawrence Weed to provide medical students with a structured documentation format oriented around the patient's problems.[2] He believed that the narrative format was often confusing and unorganized, making it difficult to determine how the physician described and treated various patient problems.[2] The POMR became a type of documentation used mainly by physicians. In the POMR, the first page of the medical record consisted of a patient problem list. This served as the table of contents for the remainder of the medical record.

Problem-Oriented Medical Record Example #1

Date: 03/15/2017
Patient: David White
Problem 1: Decreased A/PROM left wrist
Problem 2: Decreased A/PROM left ankle
Problem 3: Decreased A/PROM left knee
Problem 4: Decreased strength left wrist
Problem 5: Decreased strength left ankle
Problem 6: Decreased strength left knee
Problem 7: Edema (L) hand and ankle
Problem 8: Decreased ambulation
Problem 9: Decreased self-care
Problem 10: Decreased home management
Problem 11: Unable to work

Subsequent entries, or those that followed the initial documentation, were organized according to each problem.

The physician discussed the management of each problem in separate entries using the following headings (see POMR Example #2):

- Subjective data: Symptomatic data provided by the patient
- Objective data: Results of the physical examination
- Impression: The practitioner's impression of the patient and that particular problem
- Treatment and therapy: Treatment or therapy provided for that particular problem on that day or session
- Immediate plans (Plan): Treatment planned for that particular problem

Problem-Oriented Medical Record Example #2

Date: 03/30/17
Patient: David White
Problem #1: Decreased A/PROM of the (L) wrist

Subjective data: Pt. reports no adverse effects from last treatment; states that the wrist and hand are moving better and he can use them better during ADLs and functional activities around the house.

Objective data: AROM (L) wrist: flexion 30°, extension 30°, UD 15°, RD 20°, supination 45°, and pronation 60° taken before treatment.

Impression: Overall A/PROM improved from the initial examination. Also showed 10° improvement in wrist flexion, extension and supination following exercise during this session.

Treatment and therapy: 3 x 10 reps AROM and PROM for flexion, extension, supination, and pronation.

Plan: Have pt. continue with HEP and RTC in 2 days for progression of exercise.

Bill Jones, PTA

Using this format, the reader can identify the patient's progress and care for each of the identified problems. Some authors reported on major advantages of the POMR at the time.[3-8] Benefits of POMR included the following:

- Provided organization and structure to the medical information
- Included a comprehensive list of the patient's problems
- Discussed each of the patient's problems separately
- Provided a specific plan for managing each of the patient's problems (ie, treatment is problem-oriented)
- Allowed a physician who is interested in a particular problem to go directly to that aspect of the note, thus improving communication among care providers
- Provided a chronological sequence of interventions for a particular problem, better outlining the problem-solving process

Regardless of the benefits outlined at the time, after looking at POMR Example #2, limitations of the POMR become apparent. First, the POMR separates, or fragments, patients according to their problems, and this might pose a problem in complex cases if a provider does not see the "whole patient."[7]

In POMR Examples #1 and #2, it is possible that a therapist working with the upper extremity might not be aware of the lower-extremity problems without reading separate chart entries. This could be very time consuming. In addition, for patients with multiple problems (as in POMR Example #2), the medical record will quickly become very long and complex, requiring an extraordinary amount of time for an individual who is managing multiple problems. If one therapist were managing this patient, there would be numerous chart entries required each visit; therefore, it has typically not been suitable for more complex rehabilitation patients.[4]

More contemporary versions of the POMR have emerged that are centered around patient problems. They often include the problem, associated goal, current status, treatment directed at the problem, and plans for future interventions. A more contemporary approach is to include all of the documentation in a single chart entry or template (Figure 4-2).

SOAP Note

The SOAP note evolved from the POMR documentation format initially provided by Weed[2] described in the preceding section. As with the POMR, the subjective section should include anything that the patient tells you pertaining to his or her injuries or problems. Subjective information can also be any information provided by the patient's family or caregivers. The objective section should include the following: (1) results of screening procedures and tests and measurements performed, (2) the patient's functional status, and (3) physical therapy interventions

Date: 03/30/2017				
Patient: David White				
Problem	Associated Goal	Current Status	Intervention	Plans
1. Pt. is unable to ascend and descend stairs.	Pt. will ascend and descend stairs with supervision and assistive device.	Pt. ascends and descends stairs with min (a) x 1 using the handrail PWB 50% (L) LE.	Ther ex: (B) LE strengthening, weight shifting on/off the (L) LE x 15 minutes, stair training x 15 minutes.	Work on (B) LE strengthening, stair training.
2. Pt. is limited in mobility including ambulation.	Ambulate 200′ with crutches with (L) UE platform PWB 50% on (L) LE independently.	Pt. ambulates 100′ with crutches with (L) UE platform PWB 50% on (L) LE with min (a) x 1 to advance walker and verbal cues for weight bearing restrictions.	Gait training x 15 minutes.	Continue to advance distance, decrease level of assistance provided.
Total time = 45 minutes				

Figure 4-2. More contemporary version of POMR.

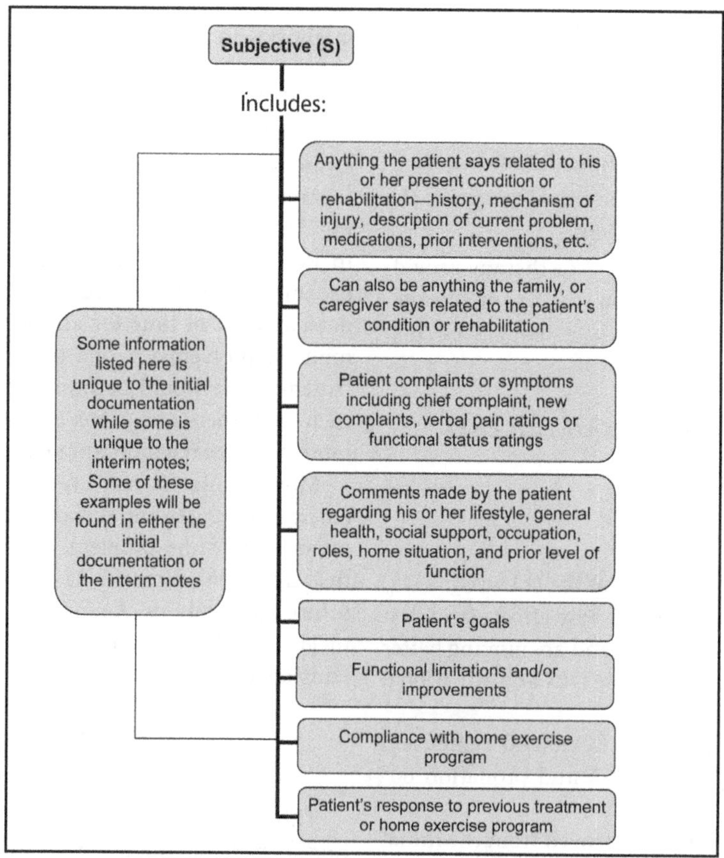

Figure 4-3. Subjective.

provided for that day of service. The interventions include procedural interventions, such as exercise and modalities, but should also include any collaboration with other disciplines and any patient or family education provided. The interpretation, or impression, has been designated A for assessment, and, in SOAP notes, the P stands for plan. Examples of information provided in the S, O, A, and P portions of initial and interim notes can be found in Figures 4-3 through 4-6.

Unlike the POMR, one SOAP note includes information pertaining to all of the patient's problems. Occasionally, the entire SOAP note is preceded by a problem (Pr) section. The

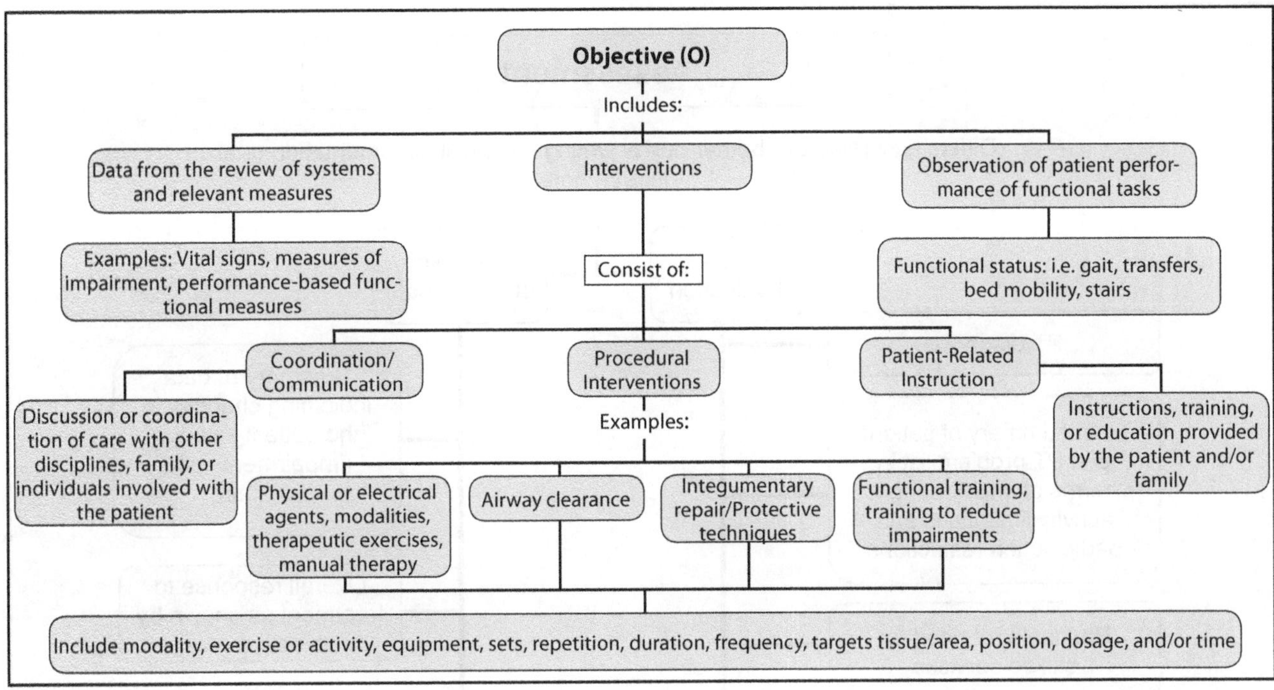

Figure 4-4. Objective.

Pr section contains information pertaining to the medical diagnosis, referral information, or information taken from the medical record (see SOAP Example later in this section). You will read more about the SOAP sections, including the Pr section, in subsequent chapters.

The SOAP format is a stand-alone format that has been widely used for some time and by a variety of medical and rehabilitation professionals. The SOAP format can be used for initial examinations and evaluations, interim documentation, and discharge documentation. The SOAP framework provides structure to medical record entries and should be used to show the clinical decision-making process in that patient/family complaints or remarks should be followed by related objective measures. Impairments, activity limitations, or participation restrictions identified in the objective data should be interpreted in the assessment, and the plan should be aimed at remediating these identified impairments, activity limitations, or participation restrictions. One contemporary modification of the SOAP note is seen in the initial documentation; the assessment and plan sections are blended into one section known as the plan of care.

SOAP Example

Date: 03/30/2017

Patient: Davis White

Pr: 27 y.o. s/p (L) wrist and ankle fx; Referral: Begin gentle wrist and ankle AROM and PROM.

S: Pt. RTC reporting no adverse effects from treatment last visit or from HEP. He stated that his wrist and ankle are moving a little better and the edema in the hand has decreased. He reports that he is able to shower (I) using a plastic chair in the tub and feels like he has improved with his ability to dress himself.

O: AROM: (L) wrist: flexion 30°, extension 30°, UD 15°, RD 20°, supination 45°, pronation 60°; (L) knee: 0–135°; (L) ankle: DF 0°, PF 45°. Girth: (L) wrist figure 8: 35.5 cm and (L) ankle figure 8: 43 cm. Tx: gentle AROM and PROM for 30' to the (L) wrist and forearm for flexion, extension, supination, and pronation; (L) ankle for DF, PF, inversion, and eversion; and for finger flexion and extension. Pt. ambulated 1000' (I) with crutches using (L) UE platform, PWB 50% on the (L) LE.

A: Pt. has made improvements in AROM and has shown decreased edema. Also reports improved function at home in ADLs, self-care, and hygiene. Gait becoming more functional and (I).

P: Will continue to have pt. perform his HEP. He will RTC 04/05/2017 for safe exercise progression within the plan of care. Will also require stair training with assistance until patient in (I) and safe.

Bill Jones, PTA

Even though SOAP notes provide a consistent and concise documentation framework, they are often criticized for being very ineffective in providing details related to the patient's need for skilled care, the patient's functional problems, or the clinician's decision-making process. Historically, there have been issues with contents of a SOAP note. First, the subjective section often contained only information about the patient's report of pain and his or her complaints. The objective section was written in terms of impairments rather than function. The assessment

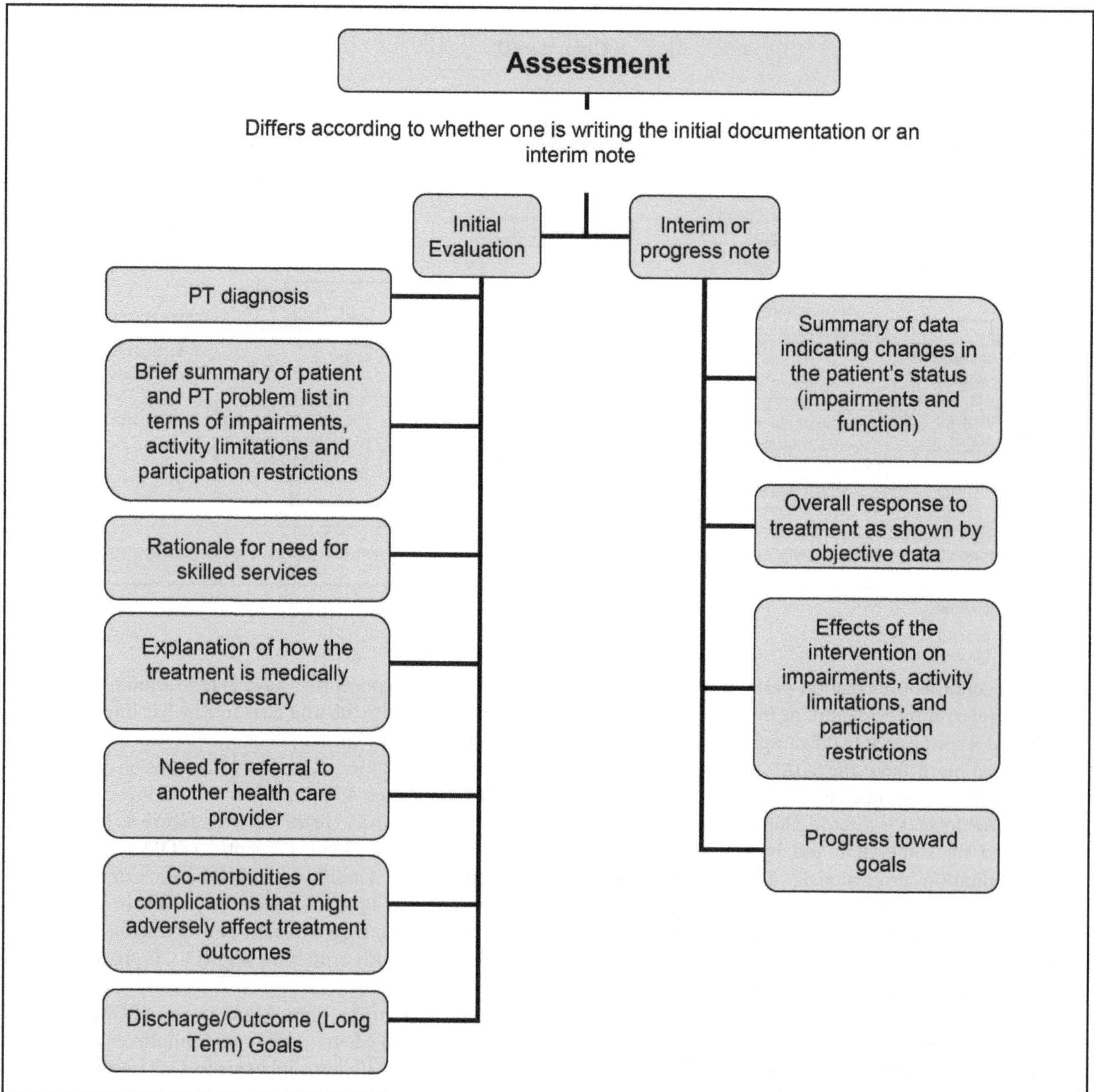

Figure 4-5. Assessment.

became a place to write a vague response to treatment, such as "tolerated treatment well," and the plan was also often written in very general terms, such as, "continue per plan." Furthermore, the relationship between impairments and functional deficits were often implied rather than overtly stated in the assessment. In addition, interventions were rarely linked to the specific impairment or functional loss at which they were aimed, and the relationship between impairment reduction and improved functional capabilities was also implied rather than described in detail in the assessment section. These problems often resulted in documentation centered around the patient's complaints and impairments, rather than his or her functional changes. Nevertheless, the SOAP format is widely known and used. It is integral to many documentation forms, templates, and electronic medical record systems. So, it is important to have a good understanding of the SOAP format components.

Functional Outcomes Reporting

The FOR is another documentation format, but its emphasis is on patient function.[1] Advantages of the FOR have been identified. The FOR clearly describes the relationship between patients' impairments and the ability to

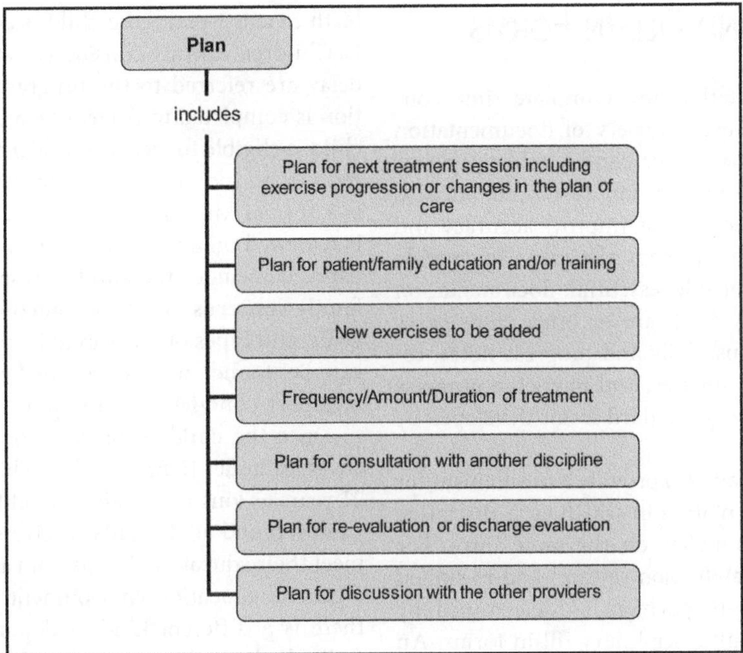

Figure 4-6. Plan.

perform functional tasks, and it improves readability for non-health care providers reviewing documentation.[1,9]

Authors have recommended integrating FOR into the SOAP structure described above by making the following additions to SOAP:

- Objective (O) section: Clearly and objectively describe the patient's functional status, including functional activities that are specific to that patient, and document his or her impairments.[9]
- Assessment (A) section: (a) List only those impairments being addressed with therapy; (b) describe how improvement in impairments will lead to improvement in function; (c) provide complicating factors, or factors that could make the duration of services longer or different from a typical case; and (d) physical therapists write goals using functional terminology.[9]
- Include the functional goal(s) at the top of daily and progress notes that were emphasized during that day of treatment (see example below).[1]

Functional Outcomes Reporting/SOAP Example

(Note: Following is the same example used to show the narrative, POMR, and SOAP formats. This example combines the FOR and SOAP formats as recommended by Abeln.[9] Additions are presented in italics.)

Goals: (1) Increase AROM in the hand, wrist, and forearm to allow (I) with ADLs, work activities, and child care. (2) Increase ankle AROM to allow normal gait pattern.

S: Pt. RTC reporting no adverse effects from treatment last visit or from HEP. He stated that his wrist and ankle are moving a little better and the edema in the hand has decreased. He reports that he is able to shower (I) using a plastic chair in the tub and feels like his ability to dress himself has improved.

O: AROM: (L) wrist: flexion 30°, extension 30°, UD 15°, RD 20°, supination 45°, pronation 60°; (L) knee: 0-135°; (L) ankle: DF 0°, PF 45°. Girth: (L) wrist figure 8: 35.5 cm and (L) ankle figure 8: 43 cm. *Functional Status: Gait: Ambulates household distances with (B) axillary crutches with (L) UE platform, PWB 50% (L), (I). Transfers: (I) with all transfers. Self-care: (I) with showering and dressing. IADLs: Unable to work; Unable to assist wife with child care duties.* Tx: gentle AROM and PROM for 30' to the (L) wrist and forearm for flexion, extension, supination, and pronation; (L) ankle for DF, PF, inversion, and eversion; and for finger flexion and extension. Pt. ambulated 1000' (I) with crutches using (L) UE platform, PWB 50% on the (L) LE.

A: Pt. has made improvements in AROM and has shown decreased edema. Also reporting improved function at home in ADLs, self-care, and hygiene. Gait becoming more functional and (I). *Decreased edema and exercise have improved AROM allowing improved use of wrist and hand during self-care and use of ankle for normal gait pattern. Continues to require use of crutches 2° to PWB status—this is limiting his ability to ambulate without an assistive device.*

P: Will continue to have pt. perform his HEP. He will RTC 04/05/2017 for safe exercise progression within the plan of care. Will also require stair training with assistance until patient in (I) and safe.

Bill Jones, PTA

Templates and Fill-In Forms

To facilitate documentation and eliminate time constraints, clinicians often use a variety of documentation templates and fill-in forms. Forms can be either paper or computer based. These forms not only save time, but also have potential to minimize writing, improve accuracy and consistency across patients, prompt clinicians to provide necessary data,[10] and include essential documentation requirements set forth by Medicare or other third-party payers.[11] Initial evaluations, daily and progress notes, re-evaluations, discharge summaries, and physician progress updates can be written using standard forms developed by individual facilities.

Forms and templates can also provide a mechanism for multidisciplinary documentation in which each discipline has its own section to complete on the same form. For example, in inpatient rehabilitation settings and in skilled nursing facilities, Medicare payment is determined by data provided through multidisciplinary fill-in forms. An example of a multidisciplinary form used in the assessment of skilled nursing facility residents is the minimum data set.[12]

While fill-in forms and templates often ease time constraints and improve consistency, both physical therapists and physical therapist assistants must take care to not allow the form to "dictate" the session. This is especially important for students and new graduates, who may feel that they cannot deviate from the form. In some instances, clinical instructors and employers will require students and new graduates to document using one of the previously described formats (ie, narrative, POMR, SOAP, FOR) rather than using the standard facility templates or fill-in forms. More important, forms can promote incomplete documentation.[9,13] Providers must be sure that forms used not only contain all essential information, but also have areas where you are able to add narrative comments.[13] These areas allow you to describe aspects of the patient's care that are not part of the standard template or form. Remember all relevant aspects of the patient's care must be documented, including characteristics unique to some patients that might not be part of the standard templates or forms. Another problem with templates is that they are often geared toward the patient population treated most at the facility. It might be difficult to use these forms when documenting on patients with less common diagnoses.

Individualized Family Service Plans and Individualized Education Plans

The Individuals with Disabilities in Education Act (IDEA) is a federal law that governs states to provide a free appropriate public education for all children with disabilities residing in the state from birth to age 21.[14] From birth to age 3 years, the child is covered under IDEA Part C. Children who are considered "at risk" for developmental delay are referred to the program, and an initial evaluation is completed to determine a child's eligibility.[15] If the child is eligible for services under this legislation, he or she receives an Individualized Family Service Plan (IFSP). This is a special kind of multidisciplinary documentation that is reviewed on an annual basis to address the needs of the child. It includes the child's present level of development, family concerns, results of outcome measures, anticipated goals, and types of services to be provided.[15] A model IFSP can be found at https://www2.ed.gov/policy/speced/reg/idea/part-c/model-form-ifsp.pdf.

Once the child turns 3, he or she may be eligible for coverage under IDEA Part B.[15] This coverage lasts until age 21 years as long as certain eligibility requirements are met. Children and adolescents receive services under Part B to meet their educational needs and allow them to function in a general education environment. Under Part B of IDEA, there is a different kind of documentation known as an Individualized Education Plan (IEP). Like the IFSP, the IEP includes the child's current academic and functional levels, a statement of his or her measurable goals, and the services that will be provided. The IEP also includes special accommodations necessary for the child to improve chances for success.[15] The IEP is also reviewed on an annual basis, at minimum. The web page http://idea.ed.gov provides resources including training for individuals involved in programs for school-aged children.[15] Physical therapy services provided to children in the school system are geared toward enhancing the child's function in the school to meet his or her educational needs. Services provided under this model are unique and differ from the medical model, where physical therapy services are most often delivered. Examples of school-based services include meeting seating and positioning needs and addressing mobility issues in and around the school. A child who is getting services in the school system under an IEP may also be receiving outpatient physical therapy to address his or her medical needs.

Both the IFSP and IEP are somewhat analogous to the physical therapist's initial plan of care in the medical model in that they serve as an outline of the expected outcomes and delineate services to be provided. Daily documentation in these settings also occurs at each encounter. In these settings, the documentation format often used is the POMR. Using this format, the physical therapist or physical therapist assistant can describe the treatment provided and the specific IEP or IFSP goal at which it is aimed.

References

1. Quinn L, Gordon J. Functional Outcomes; *Documentation for Rehabilitation*. 2rd ed. Maryland Heights, MO: Saunders Elsevier; 2010.

2. Weed LL. *Medical Records, Medical Education, and Patient Care: The Problem-Oriented Medical Record as a Basic Tool.* Chicago, IL: Year Book Medical Publishers; 1970.
3. Reinstein L, Staas WE, Marquette CH. A rehabilitation evaluation system which complements the problem-oriented medical record. *Arch Phys Med Rehabil.* 1975;56(9):396-399.
4. Reinstein L. Problem-oriented medical record: experience in 238 rehabilitation institutions. *Arch Phys Med Rehabil. 1977;58(9):398-401.*
5. Milhous RL. The problem-oriented medical record in rehabilitation management and training. *Arch Phys Med Rehabil.* 1972;53(4):182-185.
6. Mcintyre N. The problem oriented medical record. *Br Med J.* 1973;2(5866):598-600.
7. Feinstein AR. The problems of the "problem-oriented medical record". *Ann Intern Med.* 1973;78(5):751-762.
8. Dinsdale SM, Mossman PL, Gullickson G Jr, Anderson TP. The problem-oriented medical record in rehabilitation. *Arch Phys Med Rehabil.* 1970;51(8):488-492.
9. Abeln SH. Improving functional reporting (utilization review). *PT Magazine.* 1996;4(3):26, 28-30.
10. Blecker D. Building better patient notes by using templates. *ACD-ASIM Observer.* 1998;18(9).
11. Feige M. Establishing standard rehabilitation evaluation forms. Arizona Association for Home Care. *Caring.* 1992;11(8):40-44.
12. Centers for Medicare & Medicaid Services. *Minimum Data Set 3.0 public reports.* CMS.gov website. https://www.cms.gov/Research-Statistics-Data-and-Systems/Computer-Data-and-Systems/Minimum-Data-Set-3-0-Public-Reports/index.html. Updated November 14, 2012. Accessed July 9, 2017.
13. Lewis DK. Do the write thing: document everything. *PT Magazine.* 2002;10(7):30-34.
14. Individuals with Disabilities in Education Act of 2004, PL 108-446. 108th Congress (2004). http://idea.ed.gov/download/statute.html. Accessed July 9, 2017.
15. US Department of Education. *Building the legacy: IDEA 2004.* US Department of Education website. http://idea.ed.gov/. Accessed July 9, 2017.

Review Questions

1. List 4 documentation formats used in physical therapy.

2. Describe the similarities and differences between narrative notes, POMRs, SOAP notes, and FOR.

3. Describe the advantages and disadvantages of narrative notes, POMRs, SOAP notes, and FOR.

4. What type of information is found in the S, O, A, and P portions of a SOAP note?

5. When using SOAP and POMR formats, where should you place information provided by the patient's family?

6. Describe how the FOR and SOAP format can be used together.

7. What are the positive and negative aspects of using forms and templates?

8. Why is it important to learn the different documentation formats?

Application Exercises

I. Read each statement below and determine whether it would belong in the S, O, A, or P portion of a SOAP note.

1.________ Gait: Ambulated 50' x 2 WBAT (R) LE with min (A) x 1 and verbal cues to advance the (R) LE.

2.________ Pt. reports that the HEP has helped improve shoulder ROM.

3.________ Pt. will RTC for progression of his assistive device.

4.________ Transfers: bed to and from chair with mod (A) x 2.

5.________ Pt. progressing toward goals set on the initial evaluation.

6.________ Pt.'s wife stated that she has been assisting pt. with his HEP.

7.________ Speak with the PT about possible re-evaluation due to patient's rapid progress.

8.________ AROM: (R) knee 0–135°.

9.________ Improvements in knee AROM allow pt. to sit without difficulty and ascend and descend stairs with less difficulty.

10.________ Pt. feels that he is benefiting from the strengthening exercises in that he is now able to open jars and lids (I).

11.________ Pt. will be seen for bid gait training to facilitate heel strike, increased step length on the (L) and decrease fall risk.

12.________ Pt. c/o inability to move her (L) UE and LE.

13.________ Pt. denies use of assistive prior to admission.

14.________ Gait distance improved from 25' to 150' over the last week. Pt. also requiring less verbal cueing.

15.________ Pt. demonstrating (L) neglect making her unsafe during gait and transfers.

16.________ Muscle Performance: All (R) LE strength is 5/5.

17.________ Vitals: HR 95 bpm, RR 12, and BP 140/95.

18.________ Pt. has improved ability to transfer in/out of bed since initial visit from mod (a) x 1 to supervision.

19.________ Will contact PT about possible d/c evaluation as pt. is no longer benefiting from the intervention.

20.________ Pt.'s endurance is poor due to COPD.

21.________ C/O inability to brush teeth and eat with the (R) hand due to decreased AROM of the (R) elbow.

22.________ Pt. is unable to drive or perform safe community mobility at this time due to mobility and ambulation restrictions.

23.________ Edema in the (R) ankle has decreased 2 cm.

24.________ Pt. dons/doffs prosthesis (I).

25.________ Wound appearance: 100% red, healthy granulation tissue with minimal drainage.

II. Of the above statements, which would be considered "functional"?

III. Of the above statements, which link impairment to function?

IV. Your supervising physical therapist has asked you to work with a patient with the following problems: weakness in the left upper extremity, weakness in left lower extremity, dependence with ambulation, requires assist for all transfers, unable to perform self-care or home management skills.

1. List 3 questions that you could ask this patient when initiating a treatment session to elicit information for the subjective portion of a SOAP note.

2. What are 3 tests, measurements, or functional activities that you should document on this patient?

3. Compare and contrast SOAP, POMR, and FOR for this patient. What would be the same in all 3? What would be different? Which of these documentation formats would be most difficult to complete for this patient?

Chapter 5

Electronic Medical Record

Mia L. Erickson, PT, EdD, CHT, ATC

KEY TERMS Electronic health record | Electronic medical record

KEY ABBREVIATIONS EHR | EMR

Chapter Objectives

After reading this chapter, the reader will be able to do the following:

1. Explain the reason for the growth in the use of the electronic medical record (EMR).
2. Differentiate between EMR and electronic health record (EHR).
3. Describe the benefits of EMRs and EHRs.
4. Describe the barriers to implementing the electronic documentation.
5. Realize the use of electronic documentation in physical therapy.

The use of electronic patient records is growing.[1] Many physical therapists and physical therapist assistants are using computer-based documentation rather than handwriting notes in a paper-based record or using transcription. One reason for this growth is due to federal legislation that provided incentives for Medicare and Medicaid providers who were meaningfully using EHR technology.[2] As of 2015, there were penalties, or a reduction in payment, for providers who were not demonstrating meaningful use.[2] While physical therapists and physical therapist assistants are not included in these incentives and penalties, physical therapy providers who want to collaborate with physicians or health systems will be expected to use systems compatible with the Meaningful Use Program.[3] The definitions and stages for the Meaningful Use Program can be found on the Centers for Medicare & Medicaid Services website.[4]

The terms EHR and EMR are often used interchangeably; however, the differences between the 2 are significant.[5] The EMR is a digital version of the patient's chart in a hospital or clinician's office. It doesn't easily travel outside of the clinic or facility that created it, and records need to be printed for a patient to be taken to a provider outside of the clinic.[5] The EMR can take on a variety of formats. It can range from large, hospital-wide EMR systems, used by all providers in an organization, to small, individual physical therapy clinic-based systems that may or may not be connected to scheduling and billing. All systems vary in functionality, and, upon starting a job or a clinical education experience, one will need to become familiar with the EMR system used by the organization. The EHR is different. While the EHR does all of the things that the EMR does, its intention is to go beyond the clinic that collected the patient data and to allow the sharing of data between all of a patient's health providers across multiple organizations.[5]

Erickson ML, McKnight R. *Documentation Basics for the Physical Therapist Assistant, Third Edition* (pp. 41-48)

In a systematic review published in 2006, the authors reported on the benefits of EHR systems that included improved reporting, operational efficiency, interdepartmental communication, and data accuracy.[6] More recent studies have identified additional benefits including the use of EHR data for developing patient registries that can be used for research[7] and improved tracking of ancillary services and orders, legibility and accuracy, efficiency in insurance authorizations, and improved timeliness and accuracy of billing.[8] Patients also have reported the positive benefits of being able to access their medical information.[9]

Barriers to EHRs have also been identified in the literature. Vreeman et al[6] reported workflow or behavior modification, hardware or software inadequacy, and staff training as barriers to implementation. In a 2016 systematic review of literature, Kruse et al[10] reported the most frequently reported barriers, which included initial cost, technical support, technical concerns, resistance to changing work habits, maintenance/ongoing costs, and training. In another 2016 paper describing barriers to the EHR, Chan et al[11] reported similar barriers, but, in this study, the authors found that provider cooperation was the greatest barrier followed by costs and complexity of meeting Medicare's Meaningful Use Criteria. In implementing the EHR, organizations must be prepared for regularly scheduled system backups, upgrades, and maintenance of main and individual computer terminals so that there is minimal disruption to the clinical workflow. There must also be processes for storing backup files so that critical information is not lost.

The Health Insurance Portability and Accountability Act (HIPAA) provides national standards for protecting an individual's health information and for providing safeguards to maintain the security of protected health information and electronic health information.[12] HIPAA will be discussed in more detail in Chapter 12. Maintaining privacy and confidentiality of EMRs can be accomplished in several ways. For example, computer terminals should be in private areas, laptops and tablets should be held or placed where they are not viewable by patients, or privacy screen filters should be used. Computer systems maintaining patient records must be password protected with strong passwords and secured to prevent unauthorized use and assure private transmittals. They should "time out" after a brief period of nonuse.

Regardless of the security and privacy rules, data breaches occur. Data breaches can cost companies millions of dollars and can result in civil or criminal charges. The Privacy Rights Clearinghouse, a nonprofit organization that serves to empower consumers to protect their privacy, reported over 500 data breaches in the health care and medical industry in 2016 that affected nearly 4 million records.[13] Breach categories include unintended disclosure, hacking or malware, payment card fraud, insider (eg, employee, former employee), physical (eg, lost, discarded, stolen nonelectronic records), and portable device.[14]

Physical Therapy and the Electronic Medical Record

In physical therapy practice settings, using electronic documentation, the initial examinations/evaluations, daily and progress notes, re-evaluations, and discharge summaries are created using the computer documentation software. Some software packages can generate notes to the physician or case manager populated by previously recorded patient data. Physical therapy professionals log in to the software and create documentation by entering in data through templates built into the system's infrastructure. Templates are often based around body systems, regions, or pathologies. There are software packages that will allow clinicians to create their own templates around a frequently treated specific condition or patient population. Data are entered through checking boxes, selecting from a pull-down menu, or free texting into fill-in forms (Figure 5-1). Templates are often created using the SOAP (subjective, objective, assessment, and plan) format (introduced in Chapter 4), and that is why it is important to have an understanding of the SOAP contents. Figures 5-2 through 5-5 show screen shots from an EMR designed for physical therapy. Research suggests that the use of templates and standardized forms built into computerized documentation systems can help produce more complete and accurate documentation and can facilitate data mining for secondary use purposes such as research and quality reporting.[15]

Whether you are practicing at a large hospital system or a small private practice, the interface and functionality for every software package is different, and one will be required to take time to learn how to navigate the software. It is essential to understand the required elements of a good note so that, after one learns the navigation and interface, he or she will be able to input the necessary components and information. Also, one must recognize that it is difficult to capture some aspects of the episode of care in a pre-established template. For example, both medical necessity and the need for skilled care are difficult to articulate in check boxes and drop-down menus, especially when the patient is complex. There are also times when the complex patient's case does not fit easily into the computerized templates. Some information may need to be free typed into the software because of its importance. It is also important that clinicians do not get into a routine of documenting the same things for every patient, as software can prepopulate fields from previous visits and generate standard phrases. Notes can quickly start appearing the same for every visit and for every patient.

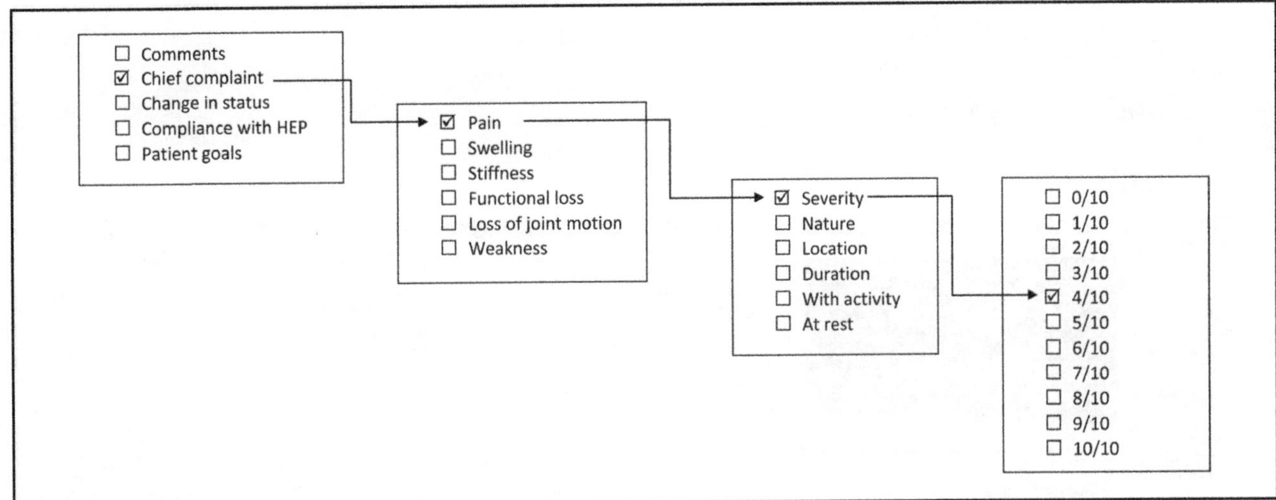

Figure 5-1. Sample electronic medical record interface.

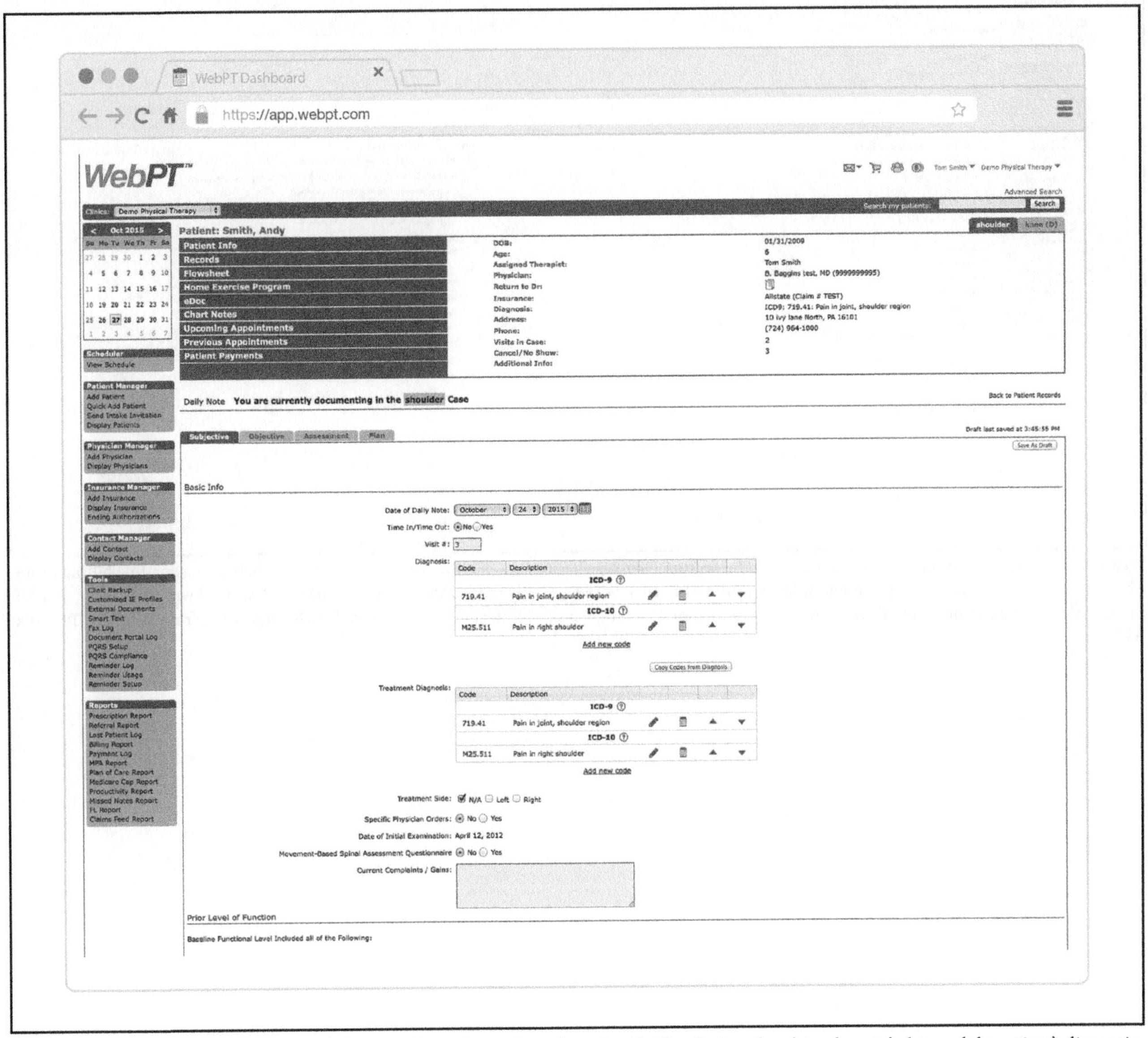

Figure 5-2. The "Subjective" tab from the daily note. This is the section where the clinician finds and updates the note's date and the patient's diagnosis, and adds subjective remarks. This information carries forward from note to note, eliminating double data entry. (Reproduced with permission from WebPT™ [Phoenix, AZ].)

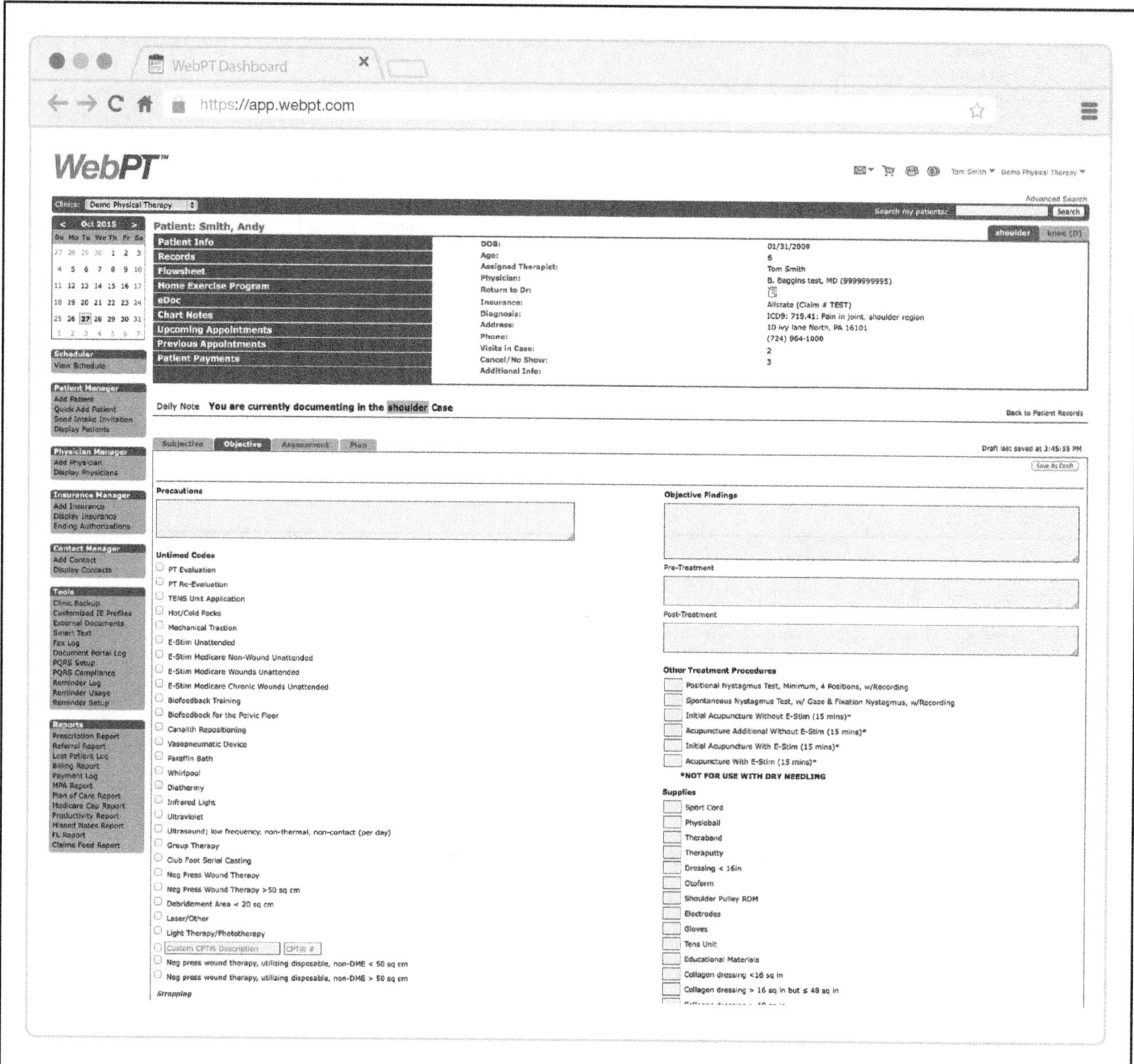

Figure 5-3. The "Objective" tab from the daily note. This section includes check boxes that link provided services to their corresponding billing codes. Those codes then automatically appear on the billing sheet associated with that daily note. Because the treatment is described within the note, you can easily make your selections and bill without having to memorize a long list of billing codes. (Reproduced with permission from WebPT™ [Phoenix, AZ].)

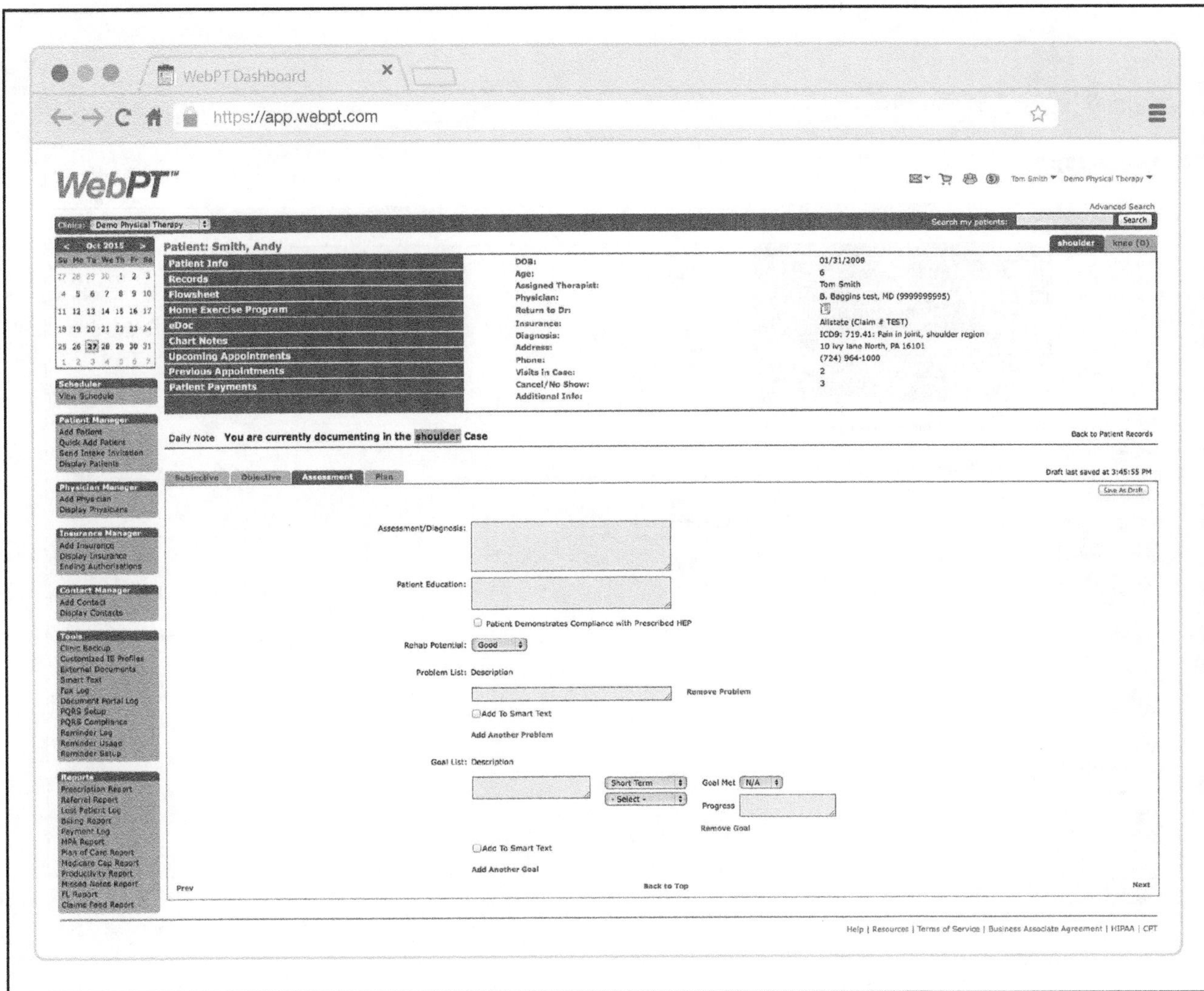

Figure 5-4. The "Assessment" tab from the daily note. One may create problems and goals that will carry forward from note to note. This makes updating progress both simple and efficient. (Reproduced with permission from WebPT™ [Phoenix, AZ].)

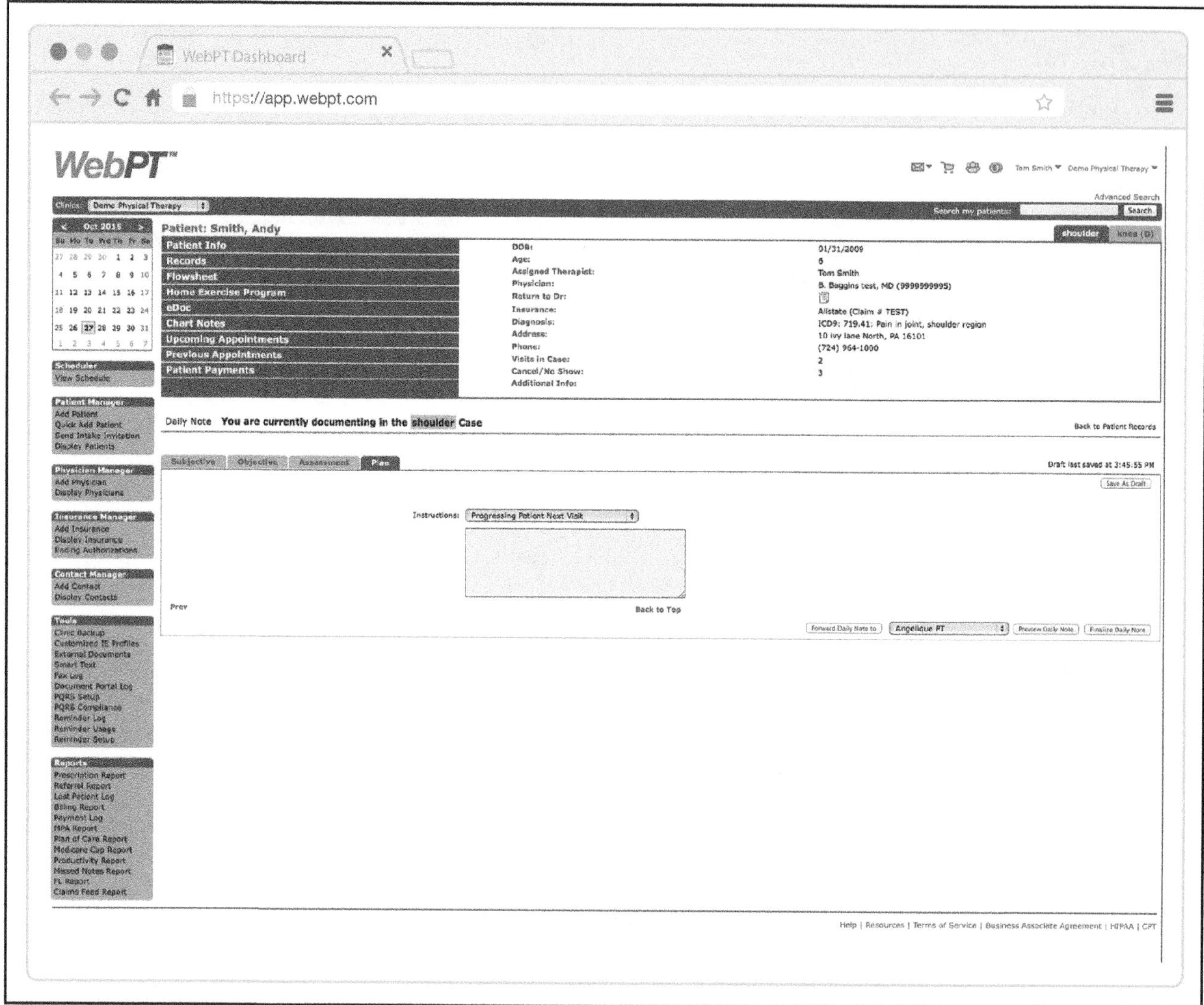

Figure 5-5. The "Plan" tab from the daily note. One selects a plan from the dropdown menu that includes commonly used treatment instructions. If more detail is needed, one then describes the plan using the expandable box below the dropdown list. (Reproduced with permission from WebPT™ [Phoenix, AZ].)

References

1. American Physical Therapy Association. *Electronic health records (EHR)*. APTA website. http://www.apta.org/EHR/. Updated May 18, 2016. Accessed July 10, 2017.
2. Centers for Medicare & Medicaid Services. *Medicare and Medicaid EHR incentive program basics*. CMS.gov website. https://www.cms.gov/regulations-and-guidance/legislation/ehrincentiveprograms/basics.html. Updated January 12, 2016. Accessed July 10, 2017.
3. American Physical Therapy Association. *Electronic health records*. APTA website. http://www.apta.org/EHR/. Updated May 18, 2016. Accessed October 16, 2017.
4. Centers for Medicare & Medicaid Services. *Electronic health records (EHR) incentive programs*. CMS.gov website. https://www.cms.gov/Regulations-and-Guidance/Legislation/EHRIncentivePrograms/index.html?redirect=/EHRincentivePrograms/. Updated June 20, 2017. Accessed July 10, 2017.
5. Garrett P, Seidman J. *EMR vs EHR—what is the difference?* Health IT Buzz website. https://www.healthit.gov/buzz-blog/electronic-health-and-medical-records/emr-vs-ehr-difference/. Updated January 4, 2011. Accessed July 10, 2017.
6. Vreeman DJ, Taggard SL, Rhine MD, Worrell TW. Evidence for electronic health record systems in physical therapy. *Phys Ther.* 2006;86(3):434-449.
7. Anderson AJ, Click B, Ramos-Rivers C, et al. Development of an inflammatory bowel disease research registry derived from observational electronic health record data for comprehensive clinical phenotyping. *Dig Dis Sci.* 2016;61:3236-3245.
8. Bobadilla JL, Roe CS, Estes P, Lackey J, Steltenkamp CL. Leveraging electronic health record implementation to facilitate clinical and operational quality improvement in an ambulatory surgical clinic. *J Ambulatory Care Manage.* 2017;40(1):9-16.
9. White H, Gillgrass L, Wood A, Peckham DG. Requirements and access needs of patients with chronic disease to their hospital electronic health record: results of a cross-sectional questionnaire survey. *BMJ Open.* 2016;6(10):e012257.
10. Kruse CS, Kristof C, Jones B, Mitchell E, Martinez A. Barriers to electronic health record adoption: a systematic review. *J Med Syst.* 2016;40(12):252.
11. Chan KS, Kharrazi H, Parikh MA, Ford EW. Assessing electronic health record implementation challenges using item response theory. *Am J Manag Care.* 2016;22(12):e409-e415.
12. Office for Civil Rights. US Department of Health & Human Services. *Summary of the HIPAA Security Rule.* https://www.hhs.gov/hipaa/for-professionals/security/laws-regulations/index.html?language=es. Accessed July 10, 2017.
13. Privacy Rights Clearinghouse. *Chronology of Data Breaches.* San Diego, CA: Privacy Rights Clearinghouse. https://www.privacyrights.org/data-breaches?title=&org_type%5B%5D=258&taxonomy_vocabulary_11_tid%5B%5D=2257. Accessed October 20, 2017.
14. Blanke SJ, McGrady E. When it comes to securing patient health information from breaches, your best medicine is a dose of prevention: a cybersecurity risk assessment checklist. *J Healthc Risk Manag.* 2016;36(1):14-24.
15. Vuokko R, Makela-Bengs P, Hypponen H, Lindqvist M, Doupi P. Impacts of structuring the electronic health record: results of a systematic literature review from the perspective of secondary use of patient data. *Int J Med Inform.* 2017;97:293-303.

Review Questions

1. Give one reason for the growth in the use of the EMR and the EHR.

2. What is the difference between the EMR and the EHR?

3. What are the benefits of the EMR and the EHR?

4. What are the barriers to implementing the EMR?

5. Describe the benefits of templates built into the EMR.

6. Describe the issues related to prepopulated fields.

7. What are positive and negative aspects of using check boxes, dropdown menus, and smart phrases?

8. Investigate Medicare's Meaningful Use Criteria. What are the stages? Provide some examples of what is required in each stage that could be relevant to physical therapy practice.

9. Research some EMR systems used in physical therapy. What are the features associated with each?

10. Interview a clinician who uses an EMR. Explore his or her opinion on the EMR and what he or she likes and dislikes. If the clinician has been part of a transition from paper to electronic records, discuss the changes that occurred in the workflow.

Chapter 6

Basic Guidelines for Documentation

Rebecca McKnight, PT, MS and Mia L. Erickson, PT, EdD, CHT, ATC

KEY TERMS Addendum | Authentication | Late entries

KEY ABBREVIATIONS APTA

Chapter Objectives

After reading this chapter, the reader will be able to do the following:

1. List components of the Patient/Client Management Model that should be documented in the medical record.
2. Identify tasks that must be documented by the physical therapist and those that can be documented by the physical therapist assistant.
3. Discuss basic principles for documentation.
4. Discuss principles for documenting patient care.
5. Correctly document late entries and appropriate correct errors in written medical records.
6. Follow appropriate guidelines when creating physical therapy documentation.

Documentation in Physical Therapy

Documentation of physical therapy services occurs over a continuum, throughout a patient's episode of care. Documentation begins with the initial examination, evaluation, and plan of care as performed and written by the physical therapist. Subsequent documentation includes interim notes for every encounter with the patient. Interim notes can be written by the physical therapist or the physical therapist assistant. Interim notes are written to record treatment sessions and serve as a record of what was billed. Progress notes are written to reflect the patient's progress toward the goals stated in the initial evaluation, as the patient's status changes, or within a required time frame as dictated by state law or third-party payers. Final documentation is performed at the summation of care. This is the last entry in a patient's record and is usually referred to as the discharge summary. This note often reflects the results of a discharge evaluation, which is also performed and written by the physical therapist. From examination to discharge, the physical therapy record should reflect the following: (1) the patient's condition or pathology; (2) impairments, activity limitations, and participation restrictions identified through appropriate tests and measurements; (3) anticipated goals and expected outcomes; (4) interventions provided, including patient education, communication with other disciplines, and specific procedural interventions; and (5) the final outcome or result of the intervention. The American Physical Therapy Association (APTA) official position on documentation states the following[1]:

Erickson ML, McKnight R. *Documentation Basics for the Physical Therapist Assistant, Third Edition* (pp. 49-57)

> Physical therapy examination, evaluation, diagnosis, prognosis, and plan of care (including interventions) shall be documented, dated, and authenticated by the physical therapist who performs the service. Interventions provided by the physical therapist or selected interventions provided by the physical therapist assistant under the direction and supervision of the physical therapist are documented, dated, and authenticated by the physical therapist or, when permissible by law, the physical therapist assistant.

In addition, the medical record should be kept in a secured file to meet confidentiality, privacy, and security requirements.

The APTA has set forth standardized *Guidelines: Physical Therapy Documentation of Patient/Client Management.*[2] These guidelines do not reflect the documentation needs of all specialty areas, but rather provide a foundation for developing more specific documentation procedures across a variety of unique and specialized settings.[2] Other authors have also reported specific guidelines for documenting in medical records.[3-10] This chapter discusses basic principles for documenting in a medical record.

Basic Principles

- **Be timely**. It is important that documentation is completed as soon after the session as possible. First, the treatment session is fresh in one's mind, and one is more likely to remember details sooner after the session rather than later. In addition, documentation will be necessary so that another physical therapist or physical therapist assistant can treat the patient in the event of an absence. There are also administrative reasons for timely documentation. These include filing reimbursement claims and sending progress updates to others involved in the patient's care, including physicians, case managers, or insurance companies. Clinics are likely to have policies in place that require the completion of all patient documentation within a given time frame.
- **Be thorough, relevant, accurate, and logical**. A reviewer should be able to examine the medical record and have an accurate, detailed portrayal of the patient and situation. Again, another physical therapist or physical therapist assistant should be able to look at the patient's record and treat the patient in the case of your absence.
- **Be clear and concise**. Although it is important to be as concise as possible, you should also still be thorough. Never leave out pertinent information for the sake of brevity.
- **Be consistent**. Use similar documentation formats throughout the patient's episode of care at your facility (eg, forms, SOAP, format, flowsheets). This makes it easy for reviewers and other health care providers to locate necessary information. Templates come built into electronic medical records and, in some software, templates can be created or loaded. Using templates can help with consistency.
- **Use objective language**. Include facts and observations. Avoid making subjective remarks about patients, including anything that cannot be substantiated by the data. This includes subjective remarks about a patient's response to a treatment (eg, "tolerated treatment well"), the patient's personality, or his or her psychological status. Also, avoid subjective terms such as appears and seems to be (eg, "patient seems depressed today").[10] Although you may be trying to provide additional information about the patient, be very careful not to make an unsubstantiated judgment, or a judgment outside of the scope of one's professional training and knowledge.[7]
- **Write legibly**. While the majority of physical therapy documentation occurs electronically, there may be instances when notes must be handwritten and they should be written legibly. Third-party payers have been known to deny claims based solely on the fact that they could not read the provider's handwriting.
- **When writing in a medical record, or creating documents that will be scanned into a medical record, use black or blue permanent ink**. Ballpoint pens are preferred over felt tip pens. Erasable ink should never be used.
- **Use scientific, medical terminology and avoid "non-skilled language."** For example, avoid statements such as, "The patient walked." Instead, use descriptive, objective, functional language that emphasizes what the patient or family member/caregiver did. For example, use statements such as the following:
  - "The patient ambulated 50' with assistance x 1 at the truck to maintain upright posture."
  - "The patient stood in the parallel bars x 2 minutes equal weightbearing on (B) LEs without loss of balance."
  - "The patient's wife was able to (I) transfer the patient from the bed to the bedside commode upon return demonstration."
  - "Upon return demonstration, the patient's caregiver was able to provide passive stretching to the patient's heel cords (I) after instruction."
- **When documenting interventions, include specific descriptions of the intervention, equipment used, number of sets, number of repetitions, treatment parameters, and any other details necessary for another therapist to recreate the session**. Flowsheets may be used as long as there is a corresponding written note describing both the skilled services provided to the patient for that day of service and the patient's response to treatment for that day of service.

- **Communicate skilled care.** Describe how the skills of the therapist were used to assist the patient. Use specific language to allow the reader to understand how the therapist's special skills and training provided assistance to the patient above and beyond what could be provided by an untrained individual. A description of how the therapist's skills assisted the patient provides important information for a reviewer and provides data to support the patient's need for skilled services. The following are some examples:
  - "The patient ambulated 25' with a quad cane. The patient required min (a) x 1 for facilitation to the (R) quadriceps during the swing phase of gait and min (a) x 1 for stabilization of the (R) knee during the stance phase."
  - "The patient required instruction in safe and effective walker use during treatment so that he could maintain weightbearing restrictions and perform safe step length."
- **Use abbreviations appropriately.** Use only industry-standard and facility-approved medical terminology, symbols, and abbreviations. Do not create your own abbreviations. Also, do not overuse abbreviations or symbols. This can become confusing for the reader, especially if he or she is unfamiliar with the abbreviations. Most word processors used in EMRs prevent the use of many symbols. In addition, some abbreviations have more than one meaning (eg, PT = physical therapist and prothrombin time). In these cases, one must read the entire note to determine the context of the abbreviation so that it can be interpreted correctly. Most facilities will have policies regarding acceptable abbreviations and their use. Common abbreviations and symbols have been provided in Appendix A.
- **When handwriting an entry for a medical record, avoid skipping lines.** Do not skip lines in the middle of entries, such as in between different sections. Skipping lines could allow someone to come back at a later date and fraudulently add information.
- **Use headings.** Headings group relevant information together to indicate new sections and to designate important patient information. They often make the note easier to read, and they identify necessary information. When handwriting notes, it is important to use the same headings that were used by the physical therapist in the initial evaluation, when possible. This will help to provide consistency between the initial evaluation and the interim notes and will allow the reader to identify data in specific sections. The use of headings is often necessary in instances when the health care providers must free text their notes into a word processing area. In the EMR, headings are often prepopulated and appear on the printed version of the note.
- **Use tables when indicated.** In instances when there are great deals of data that can easily become confusing to the reader, it is appropriate to use tables, columns, or lists. Tables are valuable when documenting range of motion or strength on several joints, such as the hand. The EMR will print reports placing data in table format, where appropriate.
- **Document late entries.** After completing the documentation for a particular treatment session and placing it in the medical record, one might realize a need to document additional information about the session. The original note should never be rewritten. Instead, complete a late entry. The entry should be placed in chronological order for the date that it is written and should be identified as a "late entry" or "addendum."
- **When handwriting entries, correct errors with a single straight black line through the text.** Initial and date next to the error. Never use correction fluid in an entry for a medical record. An individual reading the note should still be able to read what was written originally (eg, "The patient ~~ambulated~~ MLE 2/18/17 transferred from the bed to the chair with min (A) x 1 to guard at the knee to prevent buckling during stance").
- **Date and authenticate all patient records.** All physical therapy records should be dated according to the day that the services were provided. Authentication is defined as "the process used to verify that an entry into the medical record is complete, accurate, and final."[2] Indications of authentication can include original written signatures or electronic signatures. Signatures should also include the clinician's full name and designation (PT or PTA).[5]
- **Document missed appointments.** Document reasons for cancelled or missed appointments or treatment sessions, whether initiated by the patient, the physical therapist, the physical therapist assistant, or another health care provider.
  - Example 1:

    In an outpatient clinic, a snow storm in January caused your patient to miss 2 appointments. Document:
    - 1/19/17—Pt. canceled appt. due to weather, rescheduled for 1/21/17. Sue Brooks, PTA
    - 1/21/17—Pt. canceled appt. due to weather rescheduled for 1/23/17. Sue Brooks, PTA
  - Example 2:

    On a skilled nursing unit, the nurse asks that you not work with a patient because the physician suspects that the patient has a "blood clot" and is awaiting a Doppler study. Document:
    - 12/12/17—Attempted to see Mrs. Smith this am; however, nursing asked that we hold therapy 2° to possible DVT, awaiting Doppler. Will resume when cleared. Sue Brooks, PTA

- **Document telephone, face-to-face, or e-mail conversations related to patient care.** This could include conversations with the patent, the patient's family, the physician, other health care providers, or case managers.
- **Document unusual or unexpected situations or results.** Some of these situations may also require the completion of an incident report. (The completion of incident reports will be discussed further in Chapter 12 within the discussion of legal aspects of documentation.) For example, you are working with a 22-year-old woman who underwent an anterior cruciate ligament repair. She is performing resisted knee flexion with a pulley system and feels a "pop" in her knee with a moderate increase in pain.
- **When handwriting notes, indicate "continued" when using more than one page.** When the documentation of patient care requires more than 1 written page, make sure that each page includes the patient's name, the patient's medical record number, and the date. You should transition the information by writing a statement such as, "PT note for [patient's name and date] continued next page," or "PT note for [patient's name and date] continued from previous page."

Documenting Patient Care

- **Record the patient's comments using terms provided by the patient and include changes in status.** It is important to record the patient's perceptions of how the intervention is bringing about change and the relevant changes in function that he or she has noticed. For example, one may record the following: "The patient states that his exercises have helped in improving knee motion, and he is noticing improvement in sitting and ascending/descending stairs as a result."
- **Integrate disablement.** Use common, professional terminology consistent with the *International Classification of Functioning, Disability and Health Framework*.[11] Perform relevant tests and measures that are consistent with the initial examination, and record the patient's status in terms of impairments, activity limitations, and participation restrictions. Describe how the impairments are leading to activity limitations and participation restrictions. For example, one may record the following: "The patient's decreased elbow flexion is limiting his ability to brush his hair, brush his teeth, and feed himself."
- **Make comparisons between data collected at interim visits with data collected at the initial visit.** Also, make comparisons between data collected at the beginning of a treatment session and data collected at the conclusion of the session. This can help to show patient progress and the need for further intervention.
- **When documenting planned interventions, document the rationale.** For example, one may record the following: "Plan to implement electrical stimulation at the next visit to increase activity of the wrist extensor muscles."
- **Document patient education.** This includes documenting any precautions, limitations, restrictions, or instructions provided to the patient. Also, as a rule, document the patient's response or how the patient portrayed an understanding of the instructions provided. One may document the following, "After reviewing total hip precautions, the patient was able to recite them without correction, and the patient verbalized understanding."
- **Document so that the notes are in compliance with the state's Physical therapy practice act.** Upon licensure, review the practice act to identify any specific requirements related to documentation. See http://www.apta.org/Licensure/StatePracticeActs/ for a list of practice acts by state.
- **Document planned interventions without being repetitive.** One should not use the phrase "continue per plan" for multiple subsequent visits, but instead should be specific as to what skilled intervention will be provided at the next visit. Documenting the same information in the plan on several notes is received as being repetitive. It may also trigger an audit to determine if care is reasonable and necessary.

References

1. American Physical Therapy Association. *Documentation Authority for Physical Therapy Services*. HOD P05-07-09-03. https://www.apta.org/uploadedFiles/APTAorg/About_Us/Policies/HOD/Practice/Documentation.pdf. Updated December 14, 2009. Accessed November 14, 2016.
2. American Physical Therapy Association. *Guidelines: Physical Therapy Documentation of Patient/Client Management*. BOD G03-05-16-41. https://www.apta.org/uploadedFiles/APTAorg/About_Us/Policies/BOD/Practice/DocumentationPatientClientMgmt.pdf. Updated December 14, 2009. Accessed July 11, 2017.
3. Redgate N, Foto M. Pay by the rules: avoid Medicare audits and reduce payment denials with a sound strategy and proper documentation. *Physical Therapy Products*. 2003;October/November:28-30.
4. Inaba M, Jones SL. Medical documentation for third-party payers. *Phys Ther*. 1977;57(7):791-794.
5. Goode N. The reliable resource: physical therapy documentation. *PT Magazine*. 1999;7(9):30-31.
6. Lewis DK. Do the write thing: document everything. *PT Magazine*. 2002;10(7):30-34.
7. Schunk CR. Liability awareness. Advice for the new physical therapist: here are some keys to avoiding risk once you've made the transition from student to practitioner. *PT Magazine*. 2001;9(11):24-26.

8. White JA. Documentation: making it meaningful. *Physical Therapy Case Reports.* 2000;3(2):78-79.
9. Abeln SH. Liability awareness. Reporting risk check-up. *PT Magazine.* 1997;5(10):38-42.
10. Clifton DW. "Tolerated treatment well" may no longer be tolerated. *PT Magazine.* 1995;3(10):24.
11. World Health Organization. *International Classification of Functioning, Disability and Health.* Geneva, Switzerland: World Health Organization; 2001. http://apps.who.int/iris/bitstream/10665/42407/1/9241545429.pdf. Accessed July 2, 2017.

Review Questions

1. What components of the Patient/Client Management Model should be documented in the medical record?

2. What is the purpose of the APTA *Guidelines: Physical Therapy Documentation of Patient/Client Management*?

3. In a written medical record, what color ink is most appropriate?

4. A physical therapist assistant sees a patient in an acute care setting first thing in the morning. When is the most appropriate time to document the session?

5. A physical therapist documents an initial examination and evaluation using the SOAP format. In most cases, subsequent documentation should take which format?

6. How might an entry be written so that it communicates that the care the patient received is "skilled"?

7. When is it appropriate to create your own abbreviations or symbols for use in a medical record?

8. Give an example of how an error should be corrected when handwriting a note.

9. What documentation format would be appropriate to document cancellations or missed appointments?

10. How might a physical therapist assistant document patient progress? Give an example.

11. How might a physical therapist assistant integrate disablement into the patient's medical record? Give an example.

12. Give an example of a medical record entry that includes a planned intervention and a rationale.

13. When is it appropriate to document, "continue per plan"?

14. Give examples of information that a physical therapist assistant might record in the assessment section of a SOAP note.

Application Exercises

I. For the following entries, indicate examples that are inappropriate by writing an "I" next to the item. Describe why they are inappropriate.

________ Pt. walked 50'.

________ Skilled services are needed.

________ Pt. stated that she enjoys coming to PT.

________ Pt. c/o pain in the (L) knee following exercise after the last visit.

________ AROM: (R) shoulder flexion 160° abduction 120°.

________ Pt. performed QS, GS, and SLRs.

________ Pt. walked around the PT gym 2 x.

________ ROM: knee 0° to 135°.

________ Pt. is demonstrating global aphasia.

________ Pt. is demonstrating excessive hip abduction with his prosthesis during ambulation.

________ Gait: 100' with hemi walker and min (A) x 1 for trunk support and min (A) x 1 for advancing the (L) LE.

________ Transfers: bed <-> chair with min (A) x 1 due to poor balance.

________ Ther Ex: Performed 20 repetitions all exercises.

________ Bed mobility: Rolls supine <-> side lying with min (A) x 1.

________ HEP: Instructed pt. in a HEP to be performed tid.

II. Write the following information in a more clear and concise manner, as it would appear in the medical record. Include an appropriate subheading.

1. The patient walked 75 feet in the hallway of the hospital with the therapist lightly touching her back. She used a front-wheeled walker. The therapist was needed to help provide the patient with support to maintain balance.

2. The patient's strength was 3/5 for the right biceps and 4/5 for the right triceps.

3. Upon arrival to therapy, the patient told you that she had been doing her HEP without any problems and really felt like her ability to get in and out of bed has improved.

4. The patient said that her pain was 3/10 on a pain scale.

5. You performed an ultrasound to the dorsal aspect of the patient's right foot. You used 3 MHz at 50% duty cycle with the intensity set at 1.0 w/cm^2.

6. The patient demonstrated the following range of motion measurements: active range of motion for the right elbow was 130° flexion and 10° of hyperextension.

7. Knee active range of motion was 100° flexion and lacking 10° of extension.

8. The patient propelled his wheelchair around the hospital, outside on the sidewalk, and up and down several ramps with you providing verbal reminders on trunk positioning for going up and down the ramps.

9. The patient was able to put her ankle-foot orthosis on and remove it independently. She was also able to independently check her skin for any irritated areas after she removed the orthosis.

10. You instructed the patient to perform 10 repetitions of each exercise as part of her home exercise program. The exercises included ankle pumps, quadriceps setting, short arc quadriceps strengthening from 45° to 0°, and heel slides.

11. During a busy morning in a hospital, you were working with a patient who told you that she was going to be discharged and wanted home health services, primarily physical therapy. After writing the note and moving on to the next patient, you realize that you did not document the patient's desire for home therapy. What should you do? How would you document this entry into the medical record. Where should this information be placed? How might this be different if you were using an EMR?

12. When handwriting information in the medical record, you realize that you made an error in documenting the patient's AROM. It should have been 125°, not 152°. Demonstrate how to correct this mistake.

III. Organize the following information so that it is clear, concise, and suitable for entry into the medical record using the SOAP format. Indicate whether the information would fall into the S, O, A, or P portion of the note. Use subheadings where appropriate.

1. Mr. Jones comes into the clinic today and tells you that his fingers became swollen and that he has had pain at a level of 7 out of 10 since the last treatment session. He goes on to say that he has not been able to perform any of the range of motion exercises you gave him because of the incredible amount of pain he has been having. He said that he has changed his postoperative dressing once a day since the last visit, and he has had a little bit of red drainage on the bandages. He also said that he is having trouble eating and shaving due to the swelling and stiffness in the finger joints.

2. You enter Mrs. Smith's hospital room and ask her if she is ready for treatment. She agrees and tells you that she wants to be ready to walk down the aisle at her grandson's wedding without using her walker. She said that her right knee pain is not as bad as it was yesterday and she thinks that she is able to bend it more. She goes on to say that she has performed the range of motion exercises twice already this morning, and she is working on trying to get her knee to bend as much as she can. While walking using a standard walker, she asks if she can begin using a cane soon.

3. Mr. Smith comes into the physical therapy department and tells you that he notices improvement in his walking since beginning the active range of motion exercises for his ankle. He also says that he is having 0 out of 10 pain with the new exercises. He goes on to tell you that he still has pain when walking on gravel, carpet, and stairs. His job requires him to do a lot of walking on uneven terrain, and he wants to be able to do this without pain before returning to work.

4. You are assigned an inpatient who had a right cerebral vascular accident 3 weeks ago. The supervising physical therapist told you that the patient is demonstrating confusion and slurred speech, but her daughter is usually present during the sessions. Upon entering the patient's room, you notice that the daughter is not present. As you work with the patient, she tells you that she fell in the bathroom last night. She also tells you that she is afraid to get out of bed because of her fear of falling again. It was difficult for you to understand the patient due to the slurring. You also understand the patient when she says that her left shoulder is sore. While performing bedside active assistive range of motion, her daughter returns, and you comment to the daughter about the patient's fall the previous night. The daughter tells you that there wasn't a fall and that she had been there with her mother all night.

5. While treating a patient during a home health visit, the patient's son tells you that his mother (the patient) has been up all night due to left hip pain. He also tells you that he is having trouble getting his mother to walk in the house with him due to pain and fear of making her hip hurt more than it already does. He also says that he has trouble performing the range of motion exercises that you showed him during the last session. The patient tells you that, because of the pain, she feels like her hip is going to give out when she stands on it.

6. Passive range of motion measurements were as follows: Right knee flexion 100°, right knee extension 5°, hip abduction 20°, hip flexion 100°, ankle PF 20°, elbow 10° to 100°, shoulder flexion 100°, shoulder abduction 100°, hip IR 20°, ankle DF 5°, shoulder ER 60° and IR 45°.

7. The patient walked 10', twice, with 1 person supplying 25% assistance, used a standard walker, did not put any weight on the right leg, needed verbal reminders each time for placing the walker forward.

8. The patient went up and down 4 stairs with a handrail that was on the right side going up and on the left coming down; the patient used a straight cane. He required supervision from the physical therapist assistant.

9. The patient walked with the therapist at his side (but not touching him) for 100 feet, twice; vital signs before exercise were blood pressure 125/85, 15 for respirations, and 77 for heart rate; vitals after were 135/85 for blood pressure, 17 for respirations, and 87 for heart rate; the patient performed ankle pumping, elbow flexion, shoulder flexion, and knee extension for 10 repetitions before and after exercise.

10. The patient's girth at the right knee joint line was 34 cm, 2 inches above was 38 cm, 4 inches above was 42 cm, and 4 inches below was 35.5 cm. Active flexion was 120°. The patient lacked 20° of active extension. Hip and ankle active range of motion were within normal limits. Strength for the quadriceps muscle was 3-/5 and for the hamstring was 3-/5. The patient walks independently with crutches, weightbearing as much as he can tolerate on the involved extremity for 100 feet.

Chapter 7

Interpreting the Physical Therapist Initial Evaluation

Rebecca McKnight, PT, MS

KEY TERMS Documentation | Episode of care | Initial evaluation note | Record of care | SOAP note

KEY ABBREVIATIONS SOAP

CHAPTER OBJECTIVES

After reading this chapter, the reader will be able to do the following:

1. List the types of information that can be found in each component of an initial evaluation note.
2. List the questions that the physical therapist assistant should ask when reviewing the evaluation note to guide decision related to provision of selected interventions.
3. Locate and use information in the initial evaluation note to determine which interventions are to be provided and how those interventions need to be performed.
4. Locate and use information in the initial evaluation note that will assist the physical therapist assistant in judging the patient's performance and outcomes and determining what course of action needs to be taken.

It was a bright July morning. Sarah approached the outpatient physical therapy clinic with a feeling of excitement and an air of expectation. This would be her first day of patient care as a licensed physical therapist assistant. As excited as she was, Sarah was also nervous. She knew that she had an important role to play in her new position, and now she no longer had a clinical instructor or her college teachers helping her to make decisions. Questions swirled through her mind as she walked in the door. "Am I really ready for this?" "Will I remember what I learned?" Her apprehension doubled as she met with John, her supervising physical therapist. As John began to discuss with Sarah the patient care activities that he was directing her to perform that day, her questions continued to trouble her. "Will I know what to do with the patients I will be working with?" "Will the interventions I provide be effective?" "Will John have confidence in my abilities?" Sarah's anxiety followed her throughout the morning until she sat down to review the chart for her first patient, S.S. As she read the information about S.S., she realized that she knew exactly what to do, and she was able to approach her first patient that morning with confidence.

Sarah was confident as she began her day of patient care because she had a clear understanding of the physical therapy process and her role in it. Based on this understanding, Sarah knew what was expected of her, and she knew what to expect from John, her supervising physical therapist. Sarah's knowledge allowed her to be able to use the communication tool of the physical therapist initial evaluation to determine how she would proceed with S.S.'s

Erickson ML, McKnight R. *Documentation Basics for the Physical Therapist Assistant, Third Edition* (pp. 59-78)

care that day. In this chapter, we take a closer look at the physical therapist initial evaluation note. We then discuss how you, as a physical therapist assistant, will use the initial note to determine how to proceed with providing selected interventions as directed by the physical therapist.

Documentation Continuum in Physical Therapy

As noted in Chapters 2 and 6, documentation of physical therapist services should occur across the episode of care. The following 4 types of notes that may be a part of the patient's physical therapist care record: (1) initial evaluation, (2) interim notes, (3) re-evaluation, and (4) discharge summary. The only type of note that might not be found in a patient record is a re-evaluation. A re-evaluation may not be required when a patient progresses in a smooth and uninterrupted fashion within a short time frame. The other 3 types of documentation must be found in a patient's physical therapist record of care. The initial evaluation is documented at the initiation of care and includes the examination, evaluation, diagnosis, prognosis, and plan of care. Interim notes, also known as visit/encounter notes, progress notes, daily notes, or treatment notes, occur at regular intervals throughout the patient's episode of care and records intervention activities, patient's responses and progress, and any other information necessary to create a clear picture of the patient's need for and response to skilled interventions. Daily or treatment session notes should be completed by the individual providing the interventions, whether it is the physical therapist or the physical therapist. Progress notes are often summaries of the physical therapy care to date and should be completed by the physical therapist. Often, these notes are required by state law or third-party payers to ensure that the physical therapist is maintaining patient care responsibility and meeting legal and ethical expectations. Discharge notes are written at the conclusion of an episode of care and summarize the physical therapist care provided and the patient's response.

The initial evaluation note provides a clear picture of the patient by including pertinent history, risk factors, and results of tests and measures. It also includes the physical therapist's professional judgment about the patient's condition, including the diagnosis, prognosis, and anticipated goals. Finally, the evaluation note includes recommendations and the physical therapist's plan of care.

As a physical therapist assistant, you will use the physical therapist's initial evaluation note as a reference for each patient contact. The evaluation note should provide the framework upon which all patient-related activities you engage in are based. From the evaluation note, you should be able to obtain a clear picture of what is happening with the patient and how physical therapy services will be administered to address the patient's problems. You will have at least a general idea of what to anticipate when you work with the patient. This includes times when your interaction with the patient begins later in the patient's episode of care. Even though the patient might have had several physical therapy sessions, it will be important for you to review the initial evaluation note to gain a clear picture of the plan of care established by the physical therapist. In addition, you will need to review any subsequent documentation (interim and re-evaluation notes) to gain an appreciation for how the patient has responded to the interventions and to see whether there have been any updates or revisions to the plan of care.

Let's look at what a typical physical therapy evaluation note written in the SOAP (subjective, objective, assessment, and plan) note format looks like and discuss how you can utilize this information to determine what you will do with the patient. Remember, even if an evaluation note is not documented in the SOAP note format, any patient record should have the same types of information. We will use the SOAP note format as a learning tool to help you distinguish what information you need to attend to and how you need to process the information to assist in deciding how to proceed with patient care activities. Once you learn the questions that you need to ask when reviewing an evaluation note, you should be able to find the information that you need, regardless of the documentation format used.

SOAP Initial Evaluation Note

As you review a physical therapy evaluation note, you will find information related to the examination in the problem, subjective, and objective sections. Evaluation information, including the diagnosis, prognosis, and goals, can be found in the assessment portion of the note. Finally, the plan for intervention will be documented primarily within the plan section (Table 7-1). We will look at each section individually, and then discuss how you will utilize the information to make decisions about what to do during your interactions with the patient.

Problem (Pr)

As noted in Chapter 4, one adaptation to the standard SOAP format is the addition of a problem section (Pr). When included, the problem section is the first part of the initial evaluation note and provides information about the patient's reason for seeking physical therapy services. The following information may be found in this section:

- Patient's chief complaint
- Medical diagnosis
- Contraindications or precautions
- Physical therapy diagnosis
- Referral for physical therapy services
- Functional limitations
- Information gleaned from the medical record

Table 7-1

Where the Elements of the Patient/Client Management Model Can Be Found in a SOAP Note

Element of Patient/Client Management Model		SOAP Initial Evaluation Note
Examination	History	Problem
	History	Subjective
	Systems Review	Objective
	Tests and Measures	Objective
Evaluation		Assessment
Diagnosis		Assessment
Prognosis		Assessment
Prognosis		Plan
Intervention		Plan

Example 7-1

Outpatient Physical Therapy Evaluation

Patient: S.S.
Age: 32 y.o.
Date of Eval: 7/14/16
Referral: PT to eval & tx
Referring Physician: Dr. Mark Long
Pr: ICD-10: G35
 Multiple sclerosis—progressive remitting type
 Impaired motor function and sensory integrity
 Balance and coordination deficits

- Recent or past surgeries
- Past conditions or diseases
- Present conditions or diseases
- Results of medical tests

In many settings, the problem section only includes the medical diagnosis and/or referral information with the remainder listed elsewhere (Example 7-1). When a problem (Pr) section is not included, the information can be found in other areas of the patient record. Sometimes, it is a direct statement prior to the remainder of the SOAP note, which provides the reason for referral or the patient's reason for seeking physical therapy services. These umbrella statements provide the context for the remainder of the initial evaluation note.

Subjective (S)

The subjective section of a SOAP note provides all pertinent data obtained from the patient, the patient's family, or other individuals familiar with the patient's history. The subjective information is a component of the history-taking portion of the examination (Figure 7-1). The following information can be found in this section:

- Patient's current and past medical history
- Patient's symptoms or complaints
- Factors that cause the symptoms or complaints
- Patient's prior level of function
- Patient's lifestyle/occupation/societal roles
- Patient's goals

As you begin to review physical therapy documentation in a variety of settings, you will find that information gleaned from the patient's medical record can be recorded in a variety of areas. There is no standard regarding this practice. As noted previously, some information might be found in the problem or subjective areas of the note. Additionally, some settings will have a separate section labeled as "Medical History." On occasion, the information is recorded in the objective section of the note. Regardless of where the information is documented, it is important for the physical therapist to indicate when the information was gleaned from a medical record instead of a patient's self-report (Example 7-2).

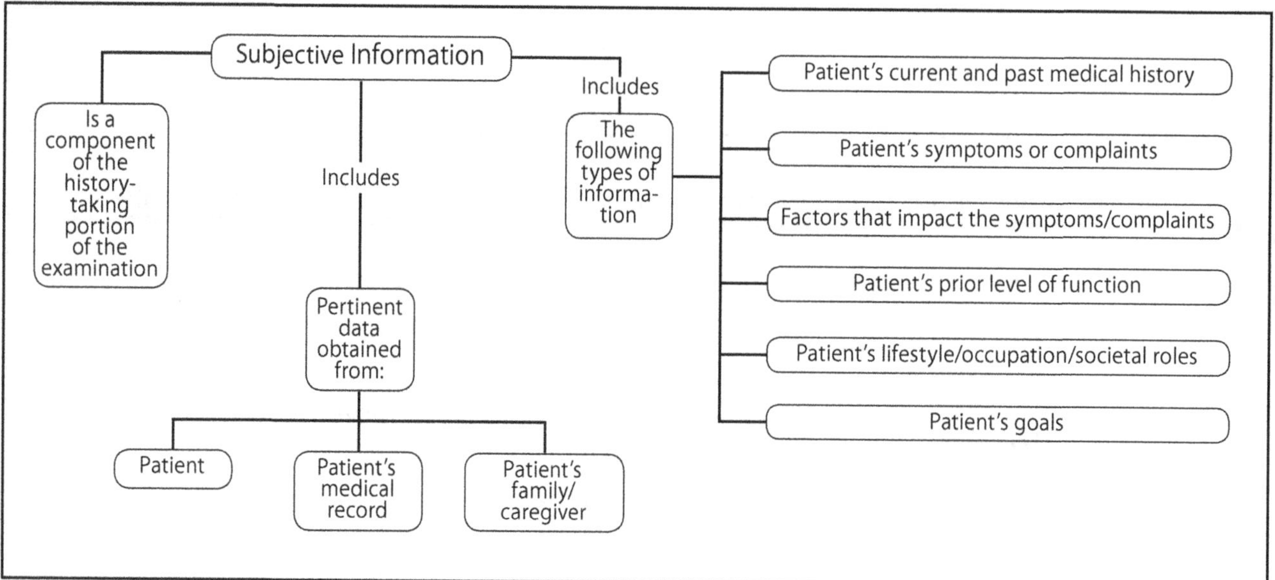

Figure 7-1. The subjective section of a SOAP note. (Reprinted with permission from Erickson M, Utzman R. McKnight R. *Physical Therapy Documentation: From Examination to Outcome*. Thorofare, NJ: SLACK Incorporated; 2012.)

Example 7-2

Subjective Component of an Initial Evaluation

S: *Demographics:* 32-year-old right-handed Caucasian female; English speaking; completed 2 years of undergraduate college education.

Social History: Pt. lives at home with her husband and 7-year-old son. Three steps with a railing to enter her one level home. Pt.'s husband works during the day and her son goes to school. Her husband has been taking time off from work to stay with her during the day, but will have to return to work this week. Pt. has various friends and family who have agreed to help during the day until she is safe to be alone at home. Pt. normally active with taking son to after-school activities.

Employment Status: She is normally employed as a bank teller, but is unable to return to work at this time due to fatigue issues and "clumsiness."

General Health Status: Pt. reports prior to this last exacerbation that she was in good health. Her primary activities included work, home care, and tending to her son, who participated in a variety of after-school activities.

Medical History: Pt. reports that she has not had any other issues that had required medical attention other than the birth of her son and typical illnesses (eg, colds, flu).

Current Condition: Pt. states that she was diagnosed with progressive MS 2 years ago. On 7/1/17 she had an exacerbation of her MS that led her to be hospitalized for 3 days of IV anti-inflammatory medications. She was discharged to home on 7/4/17 with a wheeled walker. She was receiving physical therapy while in the hospital. During her follow-up visit with her physician on 7/7/17 pt. requested more physical therapy due to balance and coordination problems. Pt. currently complains of "being unsteady on my feet," and being "clumsy with everything." Pt. reports that she will be receiving occupational therapy to address coordination problems that interfere with daily functioning.

Functional Status: Pt. states that she was previously independent with all activities of daily living and gait without an assistive device, but has been using a wheeled walker with assistance at home and a wheelchair for limited trips outside of the home due to her unsteadiness. She reports having purchased the wheeled walker from a friend at church and borrowing the wheelchair from her mother-in-law. Pt.'s

Goals: Pt. states that she would like to be able to walk without an assistive device, to return to work, and to be able to do housework.

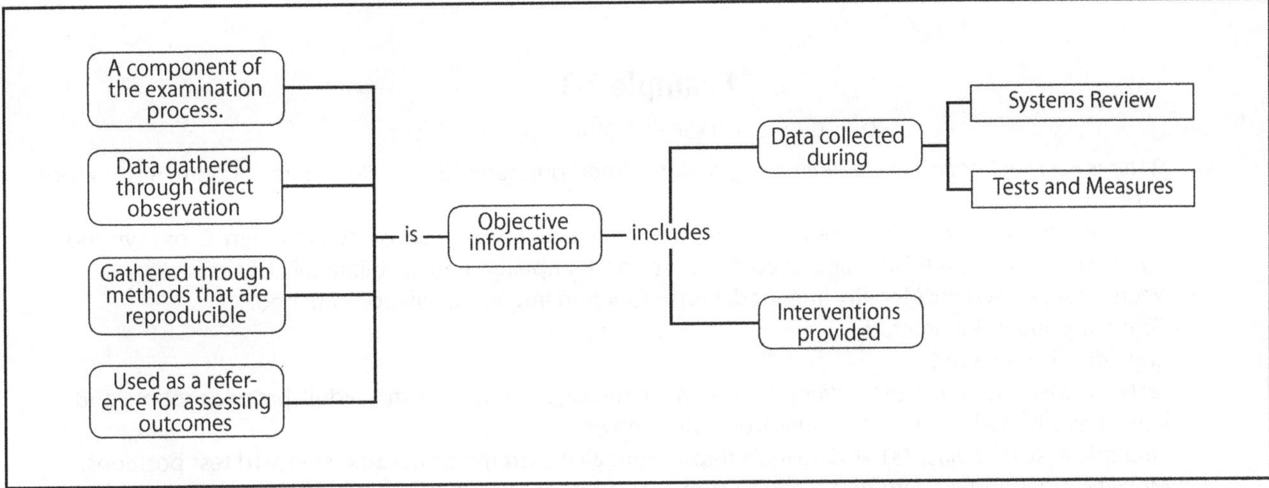

Figure 7-2. The objective section of a SOAP note. (Reprinted with permission from Erickson M, Utzman R. McKnight R. *Physical Therapy Documentation: From Examination to Outcome.* Thorofare, NJ: SLACK Incorporated; 2012.)

Objective (O)

The objective section of a SOAP note includes information gleaned during the examination via the systems review and through various test procedures, including the physical therapist's observations. Tests performed may be more diagnostic in nature, such as musculoskeletal special tests, while other tests are more prognostic in nature, such as the Berg Balance Scale, which is utilized to determine a patient's fall risk. Some tests are only appropriate for the initial evaluation, while others can be used to demonstrate the patient's progress through repeated testing throughout the episode of care. Whenever possible, the therapist should utilize standardized tests to increase the validity and reliability of the measurements obtained. Objective data must have some measure of reliability to be useful in supporting clinical decision making. In the event that a standardized test must be modified due to patient or environmental limitations, the therapist should clearly document the modifications. In addition to examination observations and measurements from tests performed, the objective section will include documentation of any interventions provided as part of the visit when the examination occurred and the patient's response to those interventions (Figure 7-2). Sidebar 2-2 in Chapter 2 lists the categories of tests and measures that can be found in the objective section of the evaluation note. As noted earlier, in addition to the data from tests, the objective section will include a category for interventions provided (Example 7-3).

Assessment (A)

The assessment section of a SOAP note documents the physical therapist's evaluation. The American Physical Therapy Association's *Guidelines: Physical Therapy Documentation of Patient/Client Management* describe evaluation as "a thought process".[1] As such, the "thought process" may not be directly documented; instead, the physical therapist will document the conclusions of the thought process. The assessment section provides an opportunity for the physical therapist to assign clinical meaning or value (evaluation) to the data collected during the examination process (documented within the subjective and objective sections of the note). The assessment section is the component of the SOAP note where the physical therapist makes a case for the need for physical therapy services by providing evidence that the services are reasonable and necessary and require the skill of a physical therapist or physical therapist. When formulating the assessment section, the therapist will sometimes choose to include a problem list that summarizes the body structure, function impairments, activity limitations, and participation restrictions. The following information may be found in the assessment section:

- Physical therapist's interpretation of subjective and objective data (an overall summary of the patient)
- Goals
- Identification of impairments in body structures and functions
- Identification of limitations in activities and participation
- The relationship between body structure and functional impairments and limitations in activities and participation
- Physical therapy diagnosis
- Prognosis/rehabilitation potential
- Justification for goals/treatment plan
- Explanation of any difficulties with obtaining subjective or objective data
- Discussion of the patient's other problems (medical, social, financial) that can impact the patient's physical functioning or participation with a plan of care (comorbidities or complexities; Example 7-4)

Example 7-3

Objective Component of Initial Evaluation

O: *Systems Review*: *Cardiovascular/Pulmonary System*: Blood pressure: 120/78. Heart rate: 78 bpm. Respiratory Rate: 16.

Integumentary System: Unimpaired; skin intact, normal pliability. Musculoskeletal System: Gross symmetry unimpaired. Gross ROM unimpaired. Gross strength impaired equally bilaterally UEs and LEs.

Neuromuscular System: Mobility impaired. Motor function impaired. Balance impaired.

Communication: Unimpaired.

Cognition: Unimpaired.

Tests and Measures and Observations: *Sensation*: Pt. displays diminished sharp/dull, proprioception, and kinesthesia in both lower extremities from knees down.

Strength: Assessed via MMT: 4-/5 to 4+/5 throughout all 4 extremities utilizing standard test positions.

Mobility: Independent with bed mobility, supine to/from sit and sit to/from stand requires standby assist to monitor pt. safety due to ataxia Pt. ambulated 200′ with wheeled walker and minimal assistance on level surfaces, demonstrating ataxia in the trunk and both legs.

Balance: Berg Balance 25.

Coordination: Pt. displays ataxia of all 4 extremities during functional tasks and during coordination tests, including finger-nose-finger and heel-shin tests.

Endurance: Fair for the above activities. Pt. stops activity due to complaints of fatigue after 15 minutes. Heart rate at time of stopping 83; Blood pressure 122/80.

Example 7-4

Assessment Component of Initial Evaluation

A: Pt.'s motor deficits, including balance, coordination, and strength deficits, prevent her from functioning independently. Pt. is unable to maintain her current employment and is not able to meet her roles as a wife and mother. Pt.'s rehab potential may be limited due to diagnosis of progressive remitting type MS. Pt.'s fatigue level will limit her participation, but, with continued efforts, pt. may be able to achieve her stated goals. Will provide a 2-week trial of physical therapy intervention to evaluate pt.'s ability to participate with physical therapy interventions and determine pt.'s potential for improvement.

Short-Term Goals: To be achieved after 2 weeks of physical therapy.

1. Independent and safe with all transfers, including supine to/from sit and sit to/from stand to allow pt. to be independent at home.
2. Pt. will ambulate with wheeled walker and standby assist on level services and minimal assistance on uneven surfaces and on stairs for walker placement and safety due to fall risk.
3. Increase general endurance so pt. can participate with 30 minutes of functional and therapeutic activities and improve independence with functional activities at home.
4. Increase strength ½ grade throughout extremities to meet the above functional goals.
5. Improve coordination of extremities to meet the above functional goals.
6. Increase balance: as evidenced by a Berg Balance Scale score of 30 to improve safety during functional activities.

Long-Term Goals: No long-term goals set at this time until potential has been assessed over the next 2 weeks of therapy intervention.

Example 7-5

Plan Component of Initial Evaluation

P: Will be seen 3 times a week as an outpatient. Pt. will receive strengthening exercises, balance, and coordination activities, functional mobility training, and gait training. Will continue gait training with wheeled walker until independent gait with wheeled walker is achieved, then will progress to gait training with other assistive device, as indicated. Will coordinate care provided with occupational therapist.

Physical therapist patient care goals should be established in conjunction with the patient and should focus on the patient's functional abilities (at the level of patient activities and participation) rather than on the level of impairments in body structures and functions. When the therapist chooses to address body structure and function impairments, it is essential for him or her to document the connections between these impairments and the patient's activity limitations and participation restrictions.

Plan (P)

The plan section of a SOAP note provides the written plan for physical therapy services and is part of the established plan of care. The following types of information may be found in the plan section:

- Plan for intervention activities, including the following:
  - Collaboration/communication with other health care providers
  - Patient-related education
  - Procedural interventions
- Frequency and duration of therapy services
- Treatment progression expectations
- Suggestions for further testing, treatment, referrals, or consultations
- Plans for further assessment or reassessment
- Equipment needs
- Referral to other services
- Anticipated discharge plans (Example 7-5)

The plan should clearly demonstrate the connection between the physical therapy interventions and the goals. When goals appropriately demonstrate the connection with the patient's activity limitations and participation restrictions, this provides a clear link between the patient's problems, the goal expectations, and the chosen interventions.

How to Use the Physical Therapist Initial Evaluation Note

When you review the initial evaluation note, you will want to glean specific information from each section to assist in determining what you need to do. To accomplish this, you need to start with a clear understanding of your role as a physical therapist assistant. As described in Chapter 2, the physical therapist assistant's role is to provide interventions as directed by the physical therapist and as outlined in the established plan of care. You will want to focus on asking questions of the evaluation note that will facilitate your ability to carry out your role efficiently. As such, the first question you should ask is, "What intervention(s) does the physical therapist want me to provide?" Answering this question first provides the appropriate context, allowing you to correctly process all other information found in the evaluation note, thus providing a proper foundation for all of the decisions you will make related to the provision of the interventions. To effectively provide the interventions, you will need to have a clear understanding of what the interventions are designed to address. Therefore, your next question should be, "What problem(s) is the intervention addressing?" For example, knowing that the physical therapist wants you to help a patient with therapeutic exercises does not give you enough information to help you determine which therapeutic exercises you will need to provide or how they need to be structured. Are the therapeutic exercises intended to address a lack of muscle strength, a cardiovascular endurance issue, or a balance deficit? The answer to this question will significantly impact how you should proceed.

After these questions have been answered, the next pair of questions you should ask will help you to determine the approach that you will take when providing the directed interventions. These questions are, "What is the patient's current status regarding impairments in body structures or functions, functional capabilities, and activity participation?" and "What are the goals set by the physical therapist and patient regarding identified problems?"

Following these questions, you should ask, "What is the patient's diagnosis?" "What is the patient's prognosis?" "Are there any contraindications or precautions that I need to keep in mind as I work with this patient?" and "Are there any other special issues that I need to keep in mind as I work with this patient?" Special issues or considerations could include things such as the patient's cognitive or psychological status. For example, it would be important to know whether the patient has a hearing or visual impairment to modify the therapy interventions to allow him or her to participate successfully in the therapy activities (Figure 7-3). The order of questions described in this section and as depicted in Figure 7-3 does not imply that one question is more important than the other. Rather, this sequence helps to ensure that the physical therapist assis-

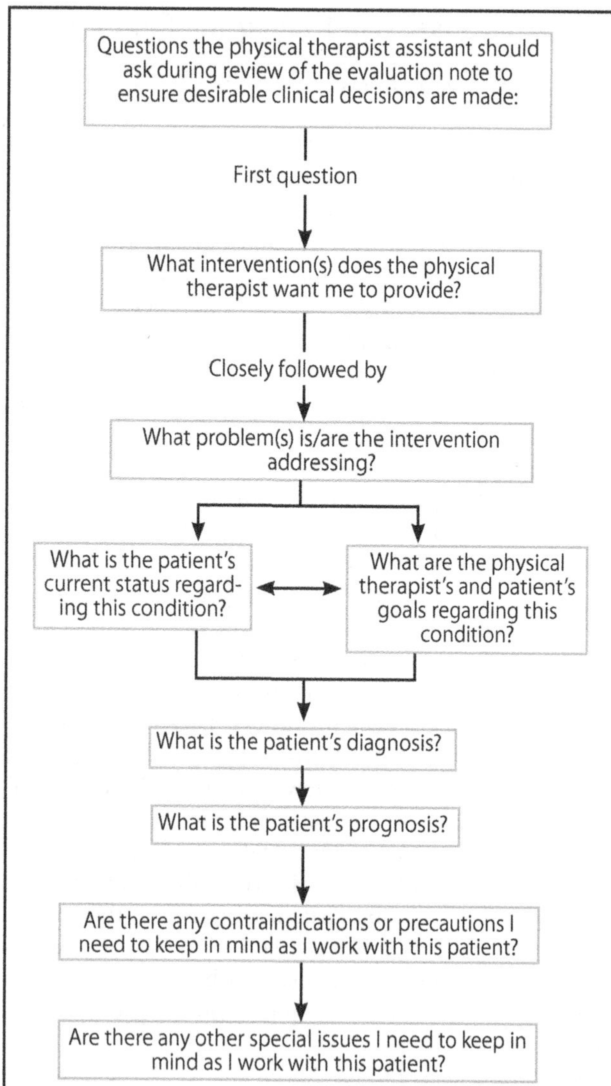

Figure 7-3. Physical therapist assistant questions for the physical therapist evaluation note.

tant is processing the information found within the evaluation note in a manner that will ensure efficient and effective clinical decision making.

Now that we have identified the questions that should guide your review of the initial documentation, let's discuss where you will find this information within the note itself.

Question 1: "What intervention(s) does the physical therapist want me to provide?"

Although this question is often answered during a direct face-to-face conversation with the physical therapist, it is important for you to review the evaluation note to discover what it says as well. On occasion, the physical therapist might ask you to perform an intervention that is not included in the plan of care. In this case, it is your responsibility to clarify the need for the intervention with the physical therapist and to ask him or her to update the plan of care accordingly. In addition, the evaluation note provides details that the therapist might not remember to communicate that can help you to determine specific strategies to utilize during patient care activities. On other occasions, you will need to determine which interventions to provide solely based on the evaluation note. To find this information, you should start by looking at the plan part of the note. In the plan section of the note, the physical therapist will have outlined the interventions to be provided. Intervention categories are listed in Chapter 2 Sidebar 2-2.

Question 2: "What problem(s) is the intervention addressing?"

As noted above, this question is imperative to help you determine, in more detail, how you will proceed when providing the intervention(s). Ideally, you will find this information in the plan alongside the intervention. For example, the physical therapist might write, "Patient to receive therapeutic exercise to address strength deficits in the right quadriceps." When this much detail is included in the plan, it is easier for you to determine how you will proceed. This level of detail helps you to quickly determine which exercises you will instruct the patient to perform. In some cases, the plan will not provide adequate information for you to determine specifically what the interventions are intended to address, or perhaps the patient has multiple areas of involvement that need to be addressed. For example, a therapist might write a broad intervention statement such as, "Patient to receive therapeutic exercises to address muscle strength and endurance issues." In this case, you will have more work cut out for you in your review to determine what muscles need strengthening.

Besides the plan section of the SOAP note, you can also find information in the assessment section (within the problem list and the goals) to help determine what problem(s) the interventions are designed to address. If, after a review of the evaluation note, you are still unclear of the purpose for the interventions, it is essential that you seek clarification from the physical therapist. Many interventions have the capacity to address more than one problem by utilizing different parameters. For example, electrotherapeutic modalities can address both pain and muscular weakness. A patient recovering from knee surgery could be dealing with both issues. If the therapist indicated the use of electrotherapeutic modalities in the plan but did not specify which problem the intervention is designed to address, you would need to clarify this prior to utilizing the modality.

When the interventions being provided focus on the level of a body structure or function impairment, it is important that you consider how these impairments impact the patient's activities and participation. Doing this ensures that you modify the intervention to address these functional issues. For example, a plan indicates that the patient is to receive strengthening exercises for weakened left knee musculature. Noting that the patient is demonstrating difficulty with going up and down stairs due to the muscle weakness can guide you to decide to focus on closed chain exercises, which more directly translate into meeting the patient's functional needs and personal goals.

Questions 3 and 4: "What is the patient's current status regarding impairments in body structures or functions, functional capabilities, and activity participation?" and "What are the goals set by the physical therapist and patient regarding identified problems?"

Information regarding the patient's current status should be reviewed considering the established goals. This will help you to get an understanding of exactly what you should expect from the patient and how you should be prepared to progress with the patient. This will also provide you with a clear expectation of how quickly the physical therapist expects the patient to progress. Information regarding the patient's current status can be found in the objective portion of the note. Further insights regarding the patient's current status can be gleaned from the problem list and the narrative, or summary statement, found in the assessment portion. Goals established by the physical therapist are listed in the assessment section of the note with clearly detailed expected timelines for reaching the goals. As noted previously, you should make sure that you identify the functional goals or the connection between impairment goals and functional activities to ensure that you make sound decisions related to the implementation of interventions. In addition, it is important to cue into statements of patient desires or goals. Helping the patient to see how the activities and interventions being performed are addressing their personal goals can help to increase the patient's motivation and participation with therapy.

Questions 5 and 6: "What is the patient's diagnosis?" and "What is the patient's prognosis?"

When looking at the evaluation note to find the patient's diagnosis, you should remember to look for both the medical diagnosis (eg, cerebrovascular accident [CVA], multiple sclerosis [MS], patella fracture) and the physical therapy diagnosis. The physical therapy diagnosis is often a statement that relates impairments to function (eg, decreased left lower-extremity strength resulting in limitations in self-care activities). The medical diagnosis may also be found in the problem section of the note. The physical therapy diagnosis will, at times, be found in the problem section as well, but it should always be found within the assessment component of the note.

The prognosis should be found as a direct statement within the assessment section of the note. The prognosis will also be communicated by the goals and time frame in which the goals are to be met. This information will provide you with a general idea of what to expect from the patient. For example, in the patient case above, as soon as Sarah read that S.S. has a diagnosis of progressive remitting MS, she had a general idea of what to expect from the patient based on her knowledge of that disease process. Further information provided in the remainder of the note helped Sarah to fill in the details so that she had a clearer picture of what to expect of S.S.'s status and performance.

Questions 7 and 8: "Are there any contraindications or precautions that I need to keep in mind as I work with this patient?" and "Are there any other special issues that I need to keep in mind as I work with this patient?"

It is imperative for you to recognize and follow any contraindications and precautions. Often, these will be directed by the physician, especially when related to recovery after a surgical procedure. When a contraindication is directed by the physician, it frequently is found within the problem component of the note. Additional precautions and contraindications might be found within the assessment or plan sections of the note. At times, contraindications and precautions are not directly specified, but rather it is expected that you will know the standard contraindications or precautions associated with conditions commonly addressed with physical therapy services. For example, a patient who is recovering from a CVA has diminished muscle performance in the musculature surrounding the shoulder joint. It is expected that you will know the appropriate precautions to take to limit subluxation and potential dislocation of the joint. Therefore, when reading all components of the evaluation note, you will want to ask yourself whether there is any information that indicates specific contraindications or precautions that you need to monitor during provision of the directed interventions.

There are numerous additional issues that you might need to consider, and it is impossible to delineate all of them. The following examples demonstrate a couple of types of issues that you would need to consider:

- Upon review of the problem and subjective areas, you might find information regarding comorbidities that can impact the patient's ability to participate in the interventions that you have been directed to provide. For example, you might be asked to provide transfer training for a patient who has left-side weakness due to a recent stroke. The chart indicates that the patient has previously had a right transtibial amputation. This information will help you to adjust your plan of action when deciding how you will approach the transfer training activities.
- Psychological and emotional issues might be recorded in the therapist's note, providing you with valuable insight into specific strategies to utilize to optimize the care provided. For example, elderly individuals who have sustained injuries due to a fall incident often deal with issues related to fear of falling that can significantly impact their ability to participate and progress in physical therapy.

Because there is such a myriad of issues that can impact the provision of physical therapy, you will want to review the evaluation note for any potential issues so that you can modify the intervention strategy or your approach to increase the likelihood for success.

Additional Questions to Answer

Once you have answered the above questions, you should have a good idea of how you will proceed while working with the patient; however, there are a few more questions that you will want to ask prior to initiating the therapy session. After you have a clear picture of what interventions you will provide and how you will provide them, you will want to ask which tests need to be performed prior to initiating the interventions. Measurements are gathered prior to beginning the interventions for 2 reasons. First, you will want to ensure that the patient's status indicates that he or she is safe to participate in the specific interventions that you have been directed to provide. Second, you will want to gather any data essential to demonstrate the patient's response to the intervention being provided.

"What tests do I need to perform prior to initiating interventions to ensure that the patient is safe and able to participate in the selected intervention(s)?"

Two pieces of data that should be collected prior to initiating any therapy session are heart rate and blood pressure. These data provide insight into the patient's physiologic status and ability to safely participate in physical therapy interventions. As you review the evaluation note, you need to identify whether the patient has a history of a cardiovascular condition or is taking any medications that can alter normal cardiovascular responses. This will help you to be prepared to respond appropriately once you have gathered the patient's heart rate and blood pressure readings.

Other data might be important to gather to determine the patient's readiness to participate in the therapy session. This will be dependent upon the individual patient case. Examples include oxygenation saturation for individuals with a respiratory condition, pain ratings for individuals recovering from a musculoskeletal surgical procedure, and cognitive status for patients who have sustained a head injury due to trauma. Again, many other conditions exist that might require you to perform preintervention tests to determine the patient's ability to participate in the interventions. You will need to review the evaluation note to determine which tests that you will need to perform, observations that you need to make, or questions that you need to ask of the patient.

"What additional tests do I need to perform to demonstrate the patient's response to the intervention(s) provided and the patient's progress toward the established goals?"

Other tests you might need to perform prior to initiating the intervention include tests that provide data regarding the patient's response to the intervention(s). Sometimes this requires pre- and postmeasurements. Just as it is important to measure heart rate and blood pressure to ensure that it is safe for the patient to participate in physical therapy, baseline data are equally important to compare pre-, during, and postintervention measurements. For example, when documenting the patient's cardiovascular response to therapeutic activities, heart rate and blood pressure measurements are the best method. Pain ratings are also commonly utilized to determine the patient's response to the interventions during and after they are provided. Some interventions are directed toward pain management, and the patient's pain ratings pre- and postintervention are needed to demonstrate the effectiveness of the intervention. At other times, pain ratings are utilized to determine what the intensity of the intervention should be. The type of data needed depends upon the particular interventions being provided, the reason for the intervention, the goals, and the time frame in which goals are expected to be accomplished. You can speak to the physical therapist if you are unsure about how to gauge intervention intensity.

As you determine which tests you should perform, you will need to make a mental list of the equipment that you will need (eg, blood pressure cuff, stethoscope). In addition, as you review the subjective information, you will want to think about what questions you might want to ask the patient. In S.S.'s case, Sarah may want to ask how the assistance from friends and family has been working out.

Some tests and measures are necessary to provide information regarding the patient's immediate response to interventions and are therefore performed pre- and postintervention (and sometimes during). In other cases, tests and measures provide a longer-term view of the patient's response to interventions and progress toward stated goals. As indicated earlier, heart rate and blood pressure measurements provide an immediate feedback regarding the patient's cardiovascular response to a particular intervention. An example of measurements that provide a longer-term view of the patient's progress includes measurements of muscle strength. In the case of S.S., to monitor the patient's progress toward the established goals and responses to the interventions provided, Sarah will observe S.S.'s functional mobility status and then will need to perform manual muscle testing (MMT) and balance and coordination testing as indicated by the time frame in the goals.

"What equipment will I need to be able to provide the intervention(s)?"

A review of the objective and assessment portions of the note will help you to determine what equipment you will need to provide the intervention(s). For example, upon review of S.S.'s evaluation note, you know that, to provide gait training activities, you will want to ensure that there is a wheeled walker and gait belt available.

"What other information should I keep in mind?"

When reading the subjective portion of the note, you also want to think about other pieces of information that you should be listening for as you provide your intervention. Frequently, patients share important information days or weeks after the initial evaluation that they forgot about at the time. This information can be useful in providing a more efficient plan of care. For example, if S.S. were to share a history of a previous right arthroscopic knee surgery with occasional knee pain, Sarah would want to document this information in the patient's chart and communicate it to the supervising physical therapist. This may help to explain discrepancies in strength gains between the legs if any are noticed in future sessions.

When you review the objective information, you want to picture in your mind how the patient will look and act. This will allow you to anticipate appropriate responses to therapeutic intervention and will help you to identify inappropriate responses. As Sarah works with S.S., she will expect the patient to fatigue and will build rest breaks into the therapy session, depending upon the level of activities performed; however, Sarah will not expect any specific complaints of pain. If, for example, S.S. begins complaining of localized pain in her left ankle, Sarah would know to consult with the physical therapist.

As you read the assessment portion of the note, you will be able to mentally outline how the patient should progress. This will guide you in the day-to-day decisions about what needs to happen with the patient. A review of the plan section will tell you the anticipated duration of the episode of care. Based upon John's assessment of S.S., Sarah would not be alarmed if the patient did not show significant improvements over the course of the treatment plan.

"Do I need to know anything else?"

The final question that you need to ask yourself is, "Is there any other information that I need that is not found in the evaluation note?" If the answer is yes, then you will want to seek out the information from the appropriate source, and that source may or may not be the physical therapist. For example, you know that the patient had laboratory work done earlier in the day. You will want to review the laboratory values to determine whether it is safe for the patient to participate in therapy or whether the physical therapist needs to be contacted. It is imperative that you ask clarifying questions prior to initiating care to ensure the safety of the patient and to improve the effectiveness of care. If the patient's initiating therapist is not available, you should ask the therapist providing supervision and direction for the patient on that day.

At this point, it should be clear how important the evaluation note is in providing essential information to guide the physical therapist assistant's decision-making process regarding interventions. In addition to providing information that helps the physical therapist assistant to proceed with patient care, the evaluation note provides a clue as to what the interim note should include. Over the next three chapters we will look at each part of a SOAP note and discuss how to compile an interim note that shows clear connections with the initial evaluation.

References

1. American Physical Therapy Association. *Guidelines: Physical Therapy Documentation of Patient/Client Management.* BOD G03-05-16-41. https://www.apta.org/uploadedFiles/APTAorg/About_Us/Policies/BOD/Practice/DocumentationPatientClientMgmt.pdf. Updated December 14, 2009. Accessed July 11, 2017.
2. American Physical Therapy Association. *Guide to Physical Therapist Practice 3.0.* APTA website. http://guidetoptpractice.apta.org/content/1/SEC2.body. Updated August 1, 2014. Accessed October 24, 2016.

Application Exercises

I. Using the case examples provided in Examples 7-6 through 7-8, practice reviewing initial evaluation notes to prepare for a treatment session. Utilize the following questions outlined in this chapter:

1. What intervention(s) does the physical therapist want me to provide?
2. What problem(s) are the intervention addressing?
3. What is the patient's current status regarding impairments in body structures or functions, functional capabilities, and activity participation?
4. What are the goals set by the physical therapist and patient regarding identified problems?
5. What is the patient's diagnosis?
6. What is the patient's prognosis?
7. Are there any contraindications or precautions that I need to keep in mind as I work with this patient?
8. Are there any other special issues that I need to keep in mind as I work with this patient?
9. What tests do I need to perform prior to initiating interventions to ensure that the patient is safe and able to participate in the selected intervention(s)?
10. What additional tests do I need to perform to demonstrate the patient's response to the intervention(s) provided and the patient's progress toward the established goals?
11. What equipment will I need to be able to provide the intervention(s)?
12. What other information should I keep in mind?
13. Do I need to know anything else?

Example 7-6

Anytown Community Hospital: Skilled Nursing Facility

Physical Therapy Evaluation
Patient: J.M.
Age: 76 y.o.
Date: 04/04/17
Referral: Physical therapy for gait and strengthening. Anterior hip precautions. Weight-bearing as tolerated.
Referring Physician: Dr. Mark John
Pr: Left total hip arthrpolasty 03/30/17. Hypertension; 2 previous TIAs approximately 1 year ago.

S: *Complaint*: Pt. states that he does have some soreness, but, in general, his hip pain is less than before the surgery; rates pain as 1–2/10 and states that it hurts worse at the end of the day.

Living Environment/Social Support: Pt. reports that he lives at home with his wife. His wife is generally in good health and is active in the community, but pt. is concerned about being a "burden" on his wife when he returns home. Pt. states that he has 3 steps with railing on 1 side to enter his one level home.

Prior Level of Function/Activities: Pt. states that he was previously independent with activities of daily living and gait without an assistive device; his hobbies include yard work and doing crossword puzzles; he is retired. Pt. normally attended church twice a week and met with friends for coffee 3-4 times a week. Pt. enjoys fly fishing 3-4 times a month "depending upon the weather."

Pt. Goals: Pt. states that he would like to return to his previous level of activity and specifically is hoping to participate in a fishing tournament this fall.

O: *Systems Review*

Cardiovascular/Pulmonary System: Unimpaired. BP: 130/85. HR: 88 bpm. RR: 20.

Integumentary System: Healing scar left hip, staples intact, no drainage noted.

Musculoskeletal System: Gross strength general decrease bilateral UEs and right lower extremity; left lower extremity impaired due to recent surgery. Gross range of motion left lower extremity restricted due to orthopedic precautions; other extremities and trunk unimpaired.

Neuromuscular System: Balance and motor control unimpaired. Functional mobility impaired.

Communication: Unimpaired.

Cognition: Unimpaired.

Tests and Measures and Observation

Strength: 4/5 to 4+/5 throughout bilateral upper extremities and right lower extremity. Left hip musculature not tested at this time due to recent surgery. Appears 2/5 with functional mobility. Left knee strength 3+/5, ankle strength 5/5.

Mobility: Scooting in bed minimal assistance to assist left lower extremity. Supine to/from sit with moderate assistance of 1, Sit to/from stand with minimal assistance of 1.

Gait: Pt. ambulated 50′ with walker and minimal assistance of one, weightbearing as tolerated left lower extremity. Pt. needed frequent verbal cues for proper walker placement due to tendency to place walker too far in front of him.

Intervention: Initiated bed mobility training, transfer training, and gait training using front wheeled walker; active assistive range of motion to left lower extremity, including ankle pumps, quad sets, ham sets, glut sets, short arc quads, straight leg raise, hip abduction, and heel slides 2 x 10. Pt. required minimal assistance of 1 with short arc quads and heel slides and moderate assistance of 1 with straight leg raises and hip abduction. Pt.

Education: Pt. was instructed in hip precautions. Pt. was able to repeat hip precautions after 10 minutes of alternate activities.

(Continued)

Example 7-6 (Continued)

A: Pt.'s decreased strength left lower extremity is limiting his functional independence. Pt. is unable to return home at this time due to dependence with mobility and need to learn hip precautions to protect recent total hip arthroplasty. This pt. is very motivated and does not have significant comorbidities and therefore has excellent rehab potential.

Problem List

1. Decreased strength left lower extremity
2. Dependent mobility
3. Dependent gait
4. Does not know hip precautions for functional tasks

Short-Term Goals: To be met within 2 days

1. Pt. will require standby to contact guard assist with all bed mobility and transfers.
2. Pt. will ambulate 100′ with walker and contact guard assist on level surfaces.
3. Increase left lower-extremity strength to 3/5 throughout hip and 4-/5 knee to be able to meet the above functional goals.
4. Pt. will be able to verbalize all hip precautions and will demonstrate understanding of precautions during basic transfers and gait activities.

Long-Term Goals: To be met within 7 days to allow pt. to return home with his wife.

1. Pt. will be independent with all bed mobility and transfers and car transfers with minimal assistanceof wife.
2. Pt. will ambulate 200′ with walker independently on level surface and up and down 3 steps utilizing railing on one side with standby assistance of wife.
3. Increase left lower-extremity strength to 3+/5 throughout hip and 4/5 knee to be able to meet the above functional goals.
4. Pt. will display good understanding of hip precautions during all functional activities, including car transfers and gait on stairs.

P: Physical therapy twice a day for ROM/strengthening exercises, transfer training including car transfers, gait training including gait on stairs and education regarding hip precautions with all functional tasks.

Ted Orlando, DPT

Example 7-7

Anytown Community Hospital: Subacute Rehabilitation

Physical Therapy Evaluation
Patient: I.H.
Pt.: Age: 68 y.o.
Date: 05/26/17
Referral: Physical therapy to evaluate and treat as advised.
Referring Physician: Dr. Sue Morton
Pr: Brainstem CVA 05/21/17, type 2 diabetes, right carotid endarterectomy 07/10, and 3 previous TIAs.

S: *Current Condition*: Pt. reports that on 05/21/17 she awoke to find that she could not get herself out of bed. She had been experiencing feelings of fatigue and weakness the evening before and had gone to bed early. Her husband called emergency services and she was transported to the hospital where the diagnosis of brainstem CVA was made. Pt.

Complaint: Pt. complains of weakness on the right side of her body and "clumsiness" with her left arm. She states she is unable to anything on her own at this point. Pt. admits to being very frustrated and just "wants to give up."

Living Environment/Social Support: Pt. reports she previously lived at home with her husband in a one-story ranch style home with one step to enter. Pt. and her husband have 3 children. One son lives in the area and can be available to assist some. The other 2 children do not live in the area. Her husband owns his own business as an electrician and will be able to cut back his "hours of work" to help her if needed.

Prior Level of Function/Activities: Pt. states she has always been a "housewife" and is sure that her husband would be unable to "run the home." Social activities include being involved in a reading club that meets monthly and going to church weekly. Pt. also reports that she occasionally keeps her neighbor's children in the evenings. The children are 5 and 8 years old.

Pt.'s Goals: She states she and her husband are hoping that she can eventually return home. She would like to return to as many of her previous activities as possible but voices she understands she may need to use a cane, walker, or wheelchair to get around. She is most concerned about being able to take care of her home including doing dishes, laundry, and general house cleaning tasks.

O: *Systems Review*

Cardiovascular/Pulmonary System: BP: 128/70. HR: 74 bpm. RR: 20

Integumentary System: Unimpaired.

Musculoskeletal System: Gross ROM unimpaired. Gross strength impaired throughout trunk and bilateral upper extremities and lower extremities right greater than left.

Neuromuscular System: Balance and motor control impaired throughout trunk and all 4 extremities. Functional mobility impaired for all tasks.

Communication: Mild slurred speech. Pt. is easily understood.

Cognition: Unimpaired.

Other: Urinary catheter noted.

(Continued)

Example 7-7 (Continued)

Tests and Measures and Observation

Observation: Pt. grossly obese.

Sensory: Pt. demonstrates normal light and gross touch, pain/thermal and diminished proprioception/kinesthesia on left and mildly diminished light and gross touch, pain/thermal, and proprioception kinesthesia on right throughout trunk and extremities.

Tone: Pt. displayed mild hypotonia right upper and lower extremity and normal tone left upper and lower extremity.

Coordination: Unable to assess right side due to weakness. Left upper and lower extremities demonstrate diminished coordination with all activities. Note apraxia and pass pointing during exercises.

Bed Mobility: Maximum assistance of 1 with rolling and scooting in bed.

Transfers: Maximum assistance of 1 supine to/from sit. Unable to perform sit to/from stand at this time. Bed to/from mat at this time is via Hoyer due to pt.'s large size, poor balance, and weakness.

MMT		Right	Left
Shoulder			
	Flexors	2/5	4/5
	Extensors	1/5	4/5
	Abductors	1/5	4/5
	Adductors	2/5	5/5
	Medial rotators	2/5	5/5
	Lateral rotators	1/5	4-/5
Elbow			
	Flexors	2/5	5/5
	Extensors	0/5	4+/5
Wrist			
	Flexors	1/5	4/5
	Extensors	0/5	4-/5
Grip		5#	28#
Hip			
	Flexors	1/5	4-/5
	Extensors	3/5	4-/5
	Abductors	0/5	4-/5
	Adductors	3+/5	5/5
Knee			
	Flexors	0/5	4/5
	Extensors	2+/5	5/5
Ankle			
	Dorsiflexors	0/5	4+/5
	Plantarflexors	1/5	5/5

(Continued)

Example 7-7 (Continued)

A: This obese pt. has very severe functional disabilities. Pt. is motivated and pleasant to work with. Due to the severe deficits, prognosis for significant recovery is poor; however, pt. and her husband want to try to get her back home. A trial of structured aggressive therapy is indicated to see how much functional return is possible for this pt. and to educate her husband on how to provide any necessary care.

Problem List

1. Decreased strength right greater than left
2. Decreased coordination left upper and lower extremities
3. Decreased balance
4. Dependent with all mobility

Short-Term Goals: Within 2 weeks pt. will display the following:

1. Moderate assist of 1 for bed mobility and supine to/from sit.
2. Maximum assist of 1 for bed to/from wheelchair using slideboard transfer.
3. Fair static and fair– dynamic sitting balance to allow for slideboard transfer goal.
4. Increase strength ½ grade throughout to be able to achieve functional goals.
5. Improve coordination left upper and lower extremity to be able to achieve functional goals.

Long-Term Goals: Within 4 weeks, pt. will display the following:

1. Minimal assistance of 1 for bed mobility and supine to/from sit.
2. Moderate assistance of 1 for bed to/from wheelchair using slideboard transfer.
3. Fair+ static and fair dynamic sitting balance to allow for transfer goals.
4. Increase strength 1 grade throughout to be able to achieve functional goals.
5. Improve coordination left upper and lower extremities to be able to achieve functional goals.
6. Pt.'s husband will safely assist her with bed mobility and all transfers.

P: Physical therapy twice a day for neuromuscular re-education, strengthening exercises, endurance activities, mobility training, and family education. Will assess pt.'s equipment needs for home use and facility acquisition of the equipment. Pt. will require, at minimum, a wheelchair and a bedside commode. Prior to discharge, recommend that pt. and her husband stay in the independent apartment to assess their ability to manage in a "home-like" environment. Anticipate continued therapy through home health services will be needed. If pt. demonstrates good recovery over her rehabilitation stay, may recommend an extension of her stay to work toward greater independence.

Joe Jackson, DPT

Example 7-8

Anytown Community Hospital: Outpatient Rehabilitation Services

Physical Therapy Evaluation

Patient: B.H.

Age: 85 y.o. Date: 09/26/17

Referral: PT for ROM and strengthening to the (L) elbow.

Referring Physician: Dr. Jeff Gordon

Pr: (L) Elbow fracture s/p ORIF 8/18/17; (L) hip fx s/p ORIF 1/15

S: *Current Condition*: Pt. states that she broke her arm when she missed a step coming out of her house into her garage 08/18/10; pt.'s husband took her to the emergency department; she had surgery the same day and returned home the next day. During a follow-up visit to the doctor on 09/21/17, the cast was removed. Pt. states that she is coming to the PT to get her "arm working again."

Patient Complaint: Pt. reports that her (L) UE seems to ache all the time especially over the weekend since her cast was removed. Pt. ranks her pain as 2/10 at rest, 3–4/10 with activities, 6–7/10 during stretching/ROM exercises. Pt. reports that she still is occasionally using painkillers prescribed by the physician and reports relief of her pain with medications.

Living Environment/Social Support: Pt. lives at home with spouse. Denies any steps to negotiate. Pt. reports prior to accident she was (I) with ADLs and gait without (A) device. Pt. does own a walker from previous (L) LE surgery; pt. reports she has needed assistance with self-care and ADLs such as bathing and dressing due to pain and stiffness since her surgery. Pt. and spouse both retired. Pt. states that she likes to garden. Pt. is (R) hand dominant.

Patient Goals: Pt. states she wants to return to her normal function.

O: *Palpation*: There is generalized soreness upon palpation of the entire (L) elbow region. Pt. also displays tenderness in the (L) brachioradialis muscle.

Inspection: Pt. displays a well-healed incision on the elbow.

ROM: (B) Shoulder AROM WNLs throughout

	(R)	(L)
PROM elbow extension/flexion	0° to 150°	90° to 130°
Forearm supination	90°	45°
Forearm pronation	90°	35°
Wrist flexion	75°	0°
Wrist extension	80°	45°

Pt. is unable to make a complete fist with the (L) hand due to discomfort and "stiffness." Formal measurements of finger joints not performed this date due to pt. needing to get to a personal function. To be deferred to next session.

Strength: (R) UE 4+/5 to 5/5 throughout all musculature. (L) shoulder 4-/5, (L) elbow pt. unable to tolerate any resistance; does perform against gravity showing 3-/5 of biceps and triceps. Grip strength (R) 40#, (L) 25#.

Intervention: pt. received MHP x 20 mins to (L) elbow and (L) hand. Gentle stretching and mobilization to elbow joints followed this. PT performed AAROM to (L) elbow, wrist and hand 10 repetitions.

Patient Education: Pt. was instructed in gentle self ROM techniques. Pt. was issued a written HEP of these ROM activities (see copy in pt. chart). Pt. was advised to use prescription pain medication approximately 30 minutes before the next therapy session to increase tolerance to the activities.

(Continued)

Example 7-8 (Continued)

A: Pt. displays limited ROM, decreased strength, and (L) hand edema, which are impeding her functional tasks at home. Pt. had an increase in pain to 6–7/10 during therapeutic ROM and stretching.

STGs: To be achieved within 5 treatment sessions. All impairment goals listed are to facilitate pt. to be able to be (I) with self-care activities.

1. Decrease edema in the (L) hand to equal the (R)
2. Increase (L) wrist ROM to WNL
3. Increase elbow flexion to 140° and extension to 0°

LTGs: To be achieved within 14 treatment sessions. All impairment goals listed are to facilitate pt. to be able to return to normal activities including house work and gardening.

1. Increase strength in the (L) elbow and hand to 4/5 to 4+/5 throughout to allow increased functional activities
2. Increase (L) elbow ROM to WNL to allow normal eating and self-care
3. Pt. will be (I) with basic ADLs and IADLs

P: Pt. to receive physical therapy 3x/week for modalities, ROM, and progressive therapeutic exercises to the (L) elbow, wrist, and hand. Will include general ROM and strengthening exercises to the shoulder to minimize effects of decreased activity on that musculature/joint.

Stephanie Wright, DPT

Review Questions

1. For each of the following components of the Patient/Client Management Model, indicate where this information can be found within an initial evaluation note written in the SOAP note format. Write Pr for problem, S for subjective, O for objective, A for assessment, and P for plan.

   ________ Prognosis

   ________ Examination: History-taking

   ________ Evaluation

   ________ Intervention

   ________ Examination: Systems review

   ________ Diagnosis

   ________ Examination: Tests and measures

2. For each of the following types of information that may be found in a physical therapy evaluation note, indicate where the information would be documented in the SOAP note format. Write Pr for problem, S for subjective, O for objective, A for assessment, and P for plan.

   ________ Rehabilitation potential

   ________ Patient education provided

   ________ Medical diagnosis

   ________ Patient's complaints

   ________ Equipment needed

   ________ Goals

   ________ Recent surgeries

   ________ Patient's prior level of function

   ________ Interventions provided

   ________ Results of tests

3. Why is it important to document patient education and communication within the intervention provided in the Patient/Client Management Model?

4. What are some questions that the physical therapist assistant should ask when reviewing the evaluation note to guide interventions?

5. Discuss the importance of starting the review of the evaluation note by determining what interventions the physical therapist wants you to provide.

Chapter 8

Writing the Subjective Section

Rebecca McKnight, PT, MS

KEY TERMS Informed consent | SOAP note | Subjective data

KEY ABBREVIATIONS SOAP

Chapter Objectives

After reading this chapter, the reader will be able to do the following:

1. List sources of information for subjective (history) data.
2. Identify types of data that should be recorded in the subjective portion of a SOAP (subjective, objective, assessment, and plan) note.
3. Discuss how subjective data are used to inform the clinical decision-making process.
4. List types of information that should be recorded in the subjection section of the interim note.
5. Describe the importance of linking subjective information in the interim note with information in the evaluation note.

Subjective data is information that the physical therapist assistant gleans from other individuals rather than data gathered through direct observation. In general terms, subjective means from the perspective of the subject or individual. As such, something is subjective when it includes the thoughts, perspectives, and emotions of the individual. The subjective section of a SOAP note contains both subjective information and simple statements of fact. For example, a patient's report of the date of his or her surgery, a nurse's report of the patient's temperature, or laboratory report finding are all information that are not filtered through a personal perspective. What makes information "subjective" for documentation in the SOAP note is not the type of information (personal perspective vs fact based), but rather the source of the information. When you include information in the subjective portion of the SOAP note, you are indicating that you obtained the information from somewhere else and did not collect the data or observe the facts yourself.

As stated, some of the information documented in the subjective section will be from a personal perspective. For example, a patient may make a statement about the impact of a condition on his or her emotional status. You might feel that information from a personal perspective is not as valuable as fact-based information; however, it is important to remember when working with people that understanding their personal perspective can be a valuable way of getting a holistic view of the person. A patient's perspective and emotions can have significant bearing on how he or she will respond to therapeutic activities, which can impact his or her progress. In this chapter, we focus on identifying the

Erickson ML, McKnight R. *Documentation Basics for the Physical Therapist Assistant, Third Edition* (pp. 79-85)

types of data that you will need to consider including in the subjective component of an interim note. Most of the time, the data will be more fact-based information. You should, however, endeavor to include patient or patient family/caregiver statements that provide insight into the patient's psychological and emotional perspective.

Where Does It Come From?

In most cases, subjective information is data gathered from the patient through direct and specific questioning. Individuals who are in close relationships with the patient may also be able to provide direct information about the patient's condition and functional status. The patient's family or caregiver can provide additional information and alternate perspectives that can help form a more comprehensive view of the patient's status. In cases where the patient has cognitive or communicative limitations and where no medical records exist, the subjective information may come entirely from the family or caregiver. In these situations, the physical therapist assistant should identify the individual who has the closest contact with the patient. This person will likely be the individual who can provide the clearest picture of the patient's functional abilities and limitations.

What Does It Include?

The subjective section of the SOAP note answers the question, "What does the patient (or the patient's family member/caregiver) have to say?" The subjective information provides the patient's perspective and documents valuable information to support the effectiveness of the treatment plan or to demonstrate the need for an alteration of the treatment plan. Subjective information includes data that provides insight into the patient's condition and its impact on the patient's functional mobility and activity participation. The physical therapist assistant should remain alert to patient and caregiver comments related to the impairments in body functions, functional limitations, and activity restrictions associated with the current condition. This information will also help the physical therapist assistant discern the patient's emotional response to these issues and will allow the physical therapist assistant to respond appropriately or modify the intervention strategies, as necessary. Specific statements, which provide a view into the patient's perspective and functional status, should be quoted within the interim note. Subjective information can provide a view into the psychosocial issues and contextual factors that influence the patient's functioning and participation.

When writing the subjective section, you should document any comments from the patient or the patient's family member(s), caregiver(s), or significant other(s) that demonstrate the following: (1) the patient's status/progress, (2) the patient's reaction to interventions provided, or (3) new problems, new complaints, or any pertinent information not previously documented. The physical therapist assistant should work to include information that provides a clear picture of how the patient is functioning.

In addition to the patient and patient's family/caregiver, a physical therapist assistant may get information about the patient from other health care providers or from a medical record. Data gathered from these sources can be recorded in several areas of the SOAP note. Regardless of where the information is documented, it is essential that the physical therapist assistant identifies the source of the information. For the purposes of the examples in this text, we record information gleaned from the medical record or received from other health care providers (eg, occupational therapist, orthotist, nurse) in the subjective component of the note. Brief, fact-based data, such as laboratory and radiologic findings, might also be documented in the problem section.

As described in Chapter 7, the initial evaluation should be a tool that you use to determine questions that you should be prepared to ask during a therapy session. As you review the initial evaluation, interim notes, and any re-evaluations, you should identify subjective data to gather that can demonstrate the patient's progress. Example 7-2 lists types of subjective information that can be found in an initial evaluation note. Two of the categories of information do not change and therefore do not need to be addressed or included in an interim note. These include general demographics and growth and development. Three of the categories contain information that is unlikely to change; however, sometimes information that the patient forgot to mention during the initial evaluation may surface in subsequent sessions or new information may surface. This includes information about the patient's medical/surgical history, family history, medications, and other clinical tests. If the patient shares information not noted in the physical therapist evaluation, you should document the information and contact the physical therapist. Likewise, you will want to document and inform the physical therapist of any new clinical test data that have the potential to impact the patient's ability to participate or progress in therapy. In the areas of social/health habits, social history, living environment, and general health status, you should note whether the physical therapist indicates a concern or issue; if so, you should be prepared to ask the patient follow-up questions related to the issue. For example, in the evaluation note, the physical therapist indicated that a patient was uncertain if he or she would go home upon discharge of if he or she would go to stay with a family member. In this case, you would want to follow up with the patient to determine if a decision had been made. As a formal review, the systems review only occurs during the initial evaluation; however, you should always be on alert and document any general issues regarding other systems that are not being addressed by the physical therapist's plan of care. For example,

Example 8-1

Problem Component of Interim Note

Anytown Community Hospital: Skilled Nursing Facility
Physical Therapy Daily Note
Patient: D.T.
Date: 04/04/16
Pr: Left patellectomy; (L) LE ROM and strength deficits; gait deficits impacting home and work life.

you might be working with a patient on lower-extremity strengthening after an orthopedic surgery when you notice a change in cognitive status that has no correlation with anything in the patient's medical record. In this case, you would document your observations and contact the physical therapist. Finally, during every patient encounter, you will need to ask questions related to the information in the areas of current condition(s), activities, and participation. You should make a mental note of the information in the initial evaluation and any interim notes to determine specific questions that you need to ask. For example, a therapist documents that a patient stated that she was unable to tie her shoes due to back pain. You should ask the patient specifically about that functional task.

Before we look at specifics about what to document in the subjective section and how to structure the note, we need to consider the problem section.

PROBLEM (PR)

You will need to record the problem prior to recording the subjective information. The problem section of the SOAP note answers the question, "What is the main problem?" In an interim note, you should document the diagnosis or main physical therapy problem. This information helps to provide a context for the rest of the documentation. You can find this information in the initial evaluation. In this section, you may also include the results of any new tests or procedures from the medical record, such as radiographs or laboratory results (Example 8-1).

SUBJECTIVE (S)

After recording the problem, you can begin to record the subjective information. As listed previously, information related to the patient's status and progress, the patient's reaction to interventions provided, and new problems or complaints should be included. Additionally, any information not previously documented that provides insight into the patient's progress should be included.

The following sections are examples of subjective information that you might need to include in the interim note.

Patient Status

Any comment that helps to paint a picture of the patient's functional status should be included. A focus should be on patient or caregiver statements that communicate the patient's ability to perform functional activities and to participate in home and community roles. Examples of information that provide insight into the patient's status include the following:

- **Pain rating and description**. For example, a 48-year-old man who is recovering from a back injury was asked to rate his pain using a numerical scale of 0 to 10 (0 = no pain and 10 = worst possible pain). The patient currently rates his pain as 3/10 and describes the pain as a "pulling" pain.
- **Patient's perception of symptoms**. For example, a 76-year-old man in a skilled nursing facility who is recovering from an exacerbation of chronic obstructive pulmonary disease reports, "I am feeling stronger."
- **Patient's functional abilities**. For example, a 35-year-old woman recovering from complications resulting from a radical mastectomy reports, "I was able to put the dishes into the cabinet last night for the first time since my surgery."
- **Statements that demonstrate the patient's cognitive or emotional status**. For example, an 84-year-old woman, recovering from an open reduction and internal fixation of a fractured femur, has been a widow for several years and was living alone prior to the accident. While in therapy, the patient states that her husband is waiting in her room to take her dancing.
- **Comments related to the accomplishment of goals/outcomes**. For example, you are working with a 32-year-old woman who is recovering from a humeral fracture. One of her personal goals is to be able to care for her 10-month-old infant. Today, in the clinic, she proudly reports, "I was able to change the baby's diaper last night all by myself."

Patient Response to Interventions Provided

- **Behavior of the patient's pain since the previous intervention**. For example, a 52-year-old woman is receiving therapy due to a diagnosis of adhesive capsulitis. The patient states that her pain level increased after her last therapy session when a new stretching activity was initiated, but she reports that the increase in pain only lasted approximately 1 hour and then the pain returned to its normal level.

- **Comments that demonstrate whether the intervention provided is effective.** For example, a 64-year-old man with chronic cervical pain has received a trial of transcutaneous electrical nerve stimulation. The patient reports no relief of pain symptoms with the transcutaneous electrical nerve stimulation trial.

New Problem(s) or New Complaint(s)

- **New pain complaints.** For example, a 77-year-old male patient is recovering from an elective total hip arthroplasty. The patient had medical complications and was on bed rest longer than anticipated, and his recovery has been delayed. As you begin working with him, he states that his heels have been very sore from lying on the bed so much.

Pertinent Information Not Previously Documented

- **Medical history.** For example, you are working in an outpatient setting. You have been assisting with the care of a 48-year-old man who injured his back while moving. Today, as you are working with him, he informs you that he had a hernia repair 2 years ago. You know that this information was not included in the initial evaluation or any of the subsequent interim notes.
- **Environment.** Lifestyle, home situation, work, school. For example, you have been assisting with the care of a 72-year-old man in a skilled nursing facility. He had a femur fracture and will be non-weighbearing for 6 to 8 weeks per the physician's report. The patient's goal is to return home, where he lives alone. You know from the evaluation note that the patient has 4 steps without any railing to enter his home. As you are working with the patient, he reveals that his "steps" are nothing more than cinder blocks stacked on top of each other.

Informed Consent

A final area that you may need to include in the subjective portion of the note is informed consent. Informed consent is a method of informing the patient of the treatment or care you will be providing. Initially, the physical therapist obtains informed consent when discussing the plan of care with the patient; however, you might be required to obtain informed consent when implementing a new modality. In this case, you are required to explain the procedure, determine the presence of contraindications, and describe risks and benefits where appropriate. You will want to record the patient's consent to the new intervention in the subjective area of the interim note.

Structure/Organization of Subjective Data

The subjective data are often highly organized in the initial evaluation note. The physical therapist will often categorize information under subheadings to provide structure to the note and to allow for a logical flow of the information. Subheadings for the information can vary and may be delineated by facility policy. When writing an interim note, subheadings are not generally necessary. You should organize the subjective information by grouping similar information. You should keep all information related to the patient's pain (rating, description, and behavior) together and keep all information related to the home environment (distance needed to walk, steps to negotiate, type of flooring) together. There may be a few occasions when you will need to document many pieces of subjective information. In this case, you can use subheadings to organize the information. When possible, use the same subheadings used by the physical therapist in the initial evaluation. Subheadings that might be used in the subjective section include the following:

- Current condition
- Patient complaint(s)
- Living environment
- Functional status/activity level
- Medical/surgical history
- Family health history
- Social history
- Employment status

Tips for Writing Subjective Information

When writing the subjective information, it is important to do the following:

- Indicate exactly who is providing the information (eg, the patient, the patient's spouse, the patient's son or daughter, the caregiver).
- Use verbs such as states, reports, complains of, denies, and describes.
- Use quotes to demonstrate the patient's cognitive or emotional status or attitude toward therapy.
- While the first word of the subjective is usually "patient," it is not necessary to repeat "patient" at the beginning of every sentence. Once it is written the first time, it is implied in subsequent sentences (Example 8-2).[1]

Example 8-2

Subjective Component of Interim Note

S: Patient complains of continued weakness in left knee. Reports being ambulatory with no assistive device when at home, uses one crutch when on uneven surfaces, outside of the home. States that he has made moderate improvements with therapy.

Reference

1. Kettenbach G. *Writing SOAP Notes.* 2nd ed. Philadelphia, PA: F.A. Davis; 1995.

Review Questions

1. What are the types of information that should be documented in the subjective portion of an interim SOAP note?

2. Identify appropriate sources for obtaining subjective information. Compare and contrast the validity of each source.

3. Indicate the preferred source (patient, patient's family member/caregiver, patient's medical chart) to obtain the following information, and describe why that is the preferred source.
   ________ Number of steps leading into the home
   ________ Description of pain
   ________ Patient's ability to get in/out of bed
   ________ Patient's prior health status
   ________ Last time pain medication was taken
   ________ Sleep patterns
   ________ Patient's adjustment to a permanent disability
   ________ Distance from the bed to the bathroom
   ________ School-related expectations for a pediatric client

Application Exercises

I. Write the following statements in a more clear and concise manner, as they would appear in the medical record. Indicate the subheading that the information would fall under.

1. The patient said that his global functional rating is 85% on a 100-point scale.

2. The patient said that he is planning to return home after he is released from the hospital.

3. The patient's wife said that the patient has not been able to get up out of bed by himself for the past 2 weeks.

4. The patient said that he has not been able to complete his work tasks because he gets tired and must sit down about every 5 minutes.

5. The patient's husband tells the physical therapist assistant that to get from the car to the house the patient must walk about 25 feet over grass and then will need to go up 4 steps and that the steps do not have a railing.

II. Organize the following information so that it is clear, concise, and suitable for entry into the medical record.

1. You are working with Mr. Jones, who injured his hand in a work accident. He complains of continued swelling in his fingers. He says that he has pain at a level of 7 out of 10 on a 10-point scale. He says that he has not been able to make a fist and that has had difficulty with getting dressed and eating due to the swelling and pain in his hand.

2. Upon seeing a child for a school-based intervention, the teacher tells you that she noticed a red spot on the arch of the child 's right foot after removing his "leg brace" (a rigid ankle-foot orthosis). She also tells you that the child is refusing to walk in the classroom and doesn't put weight on his right foot when transferring in or out of his wheelchair.

3. You are seeing a 2-year-old girl in the state's Early Intervention Program. She has a congenital right transtibial amputation. She is in foster care. During the session, the foster mom tells you that the child will be getting fit for a new prosthesis and that her doctor recommended that she go to a rehabilitation hospital to learn how to use it.

4. A 19-year-old patient is in a coma after a motor vehicle accident. The patient's mother states that the patient is a very active individual and is involved in basketball and baseball. The mother says that the patient was attending college at the local university and has been living in the dorm rooms. The mother states that the patient has been responding to her by squeezing her hand, but the patient has not said anything to her.

Chapter 9

Writing the Objective Section

Rebecca McKnight, PT, MS

KEY TERMS Evaluation note | Interim note | Objective data | Procedural interventions | SOAP note

KEY ABBREVIATIONS APTA | FIM | ROM | SOAP

Chapter Objectives

After reading this chapter, the reader will be able to do the following:

1. Identify types of data that should be recorded in the objective portion of a SOAP (subjective, objective, assessment, and plan) note.
2. Discuss how objective data are used to inform the decision related to the provision of patient care.
3. Describe documentation strategies that demonstrate that skilled care is being provided.
4. Arrange data collected during the objective portion of an interim note into a logically sequenced, objective note.
5. Describe the importance of linking objective information in the interim note with information in the evaluation note.

The objective section of a SOAP note answers the questions, "What is going on with the physical therapy intervention?" and "How is the patient responding to the intervention?" For a physical therapist (or a physical therapist assistant to utilize documentation to make appropriate decisions regarding patient care, it is essential that details regarding the interventions provided and the patient's responses to those interventions are documented. For example, if you are providing gait training with a patient who requires verbal and tactile cues, specifying details about the cues (eg, amount, location, type, frequency) can help the therapist to get a clear picture of how the patient is performing and to make appropriate decisions regarding needed modifications in the plan of care. Furthermore, these kinds of details are necessary to show that the interventions provided require the problem-solving skills of a physical therapist assistant meeting therefore meeting reimbursement requirements. The American Physical Therapy Association (APTA) *Defensible Documentation for Patient/Client Management* states the following[1]:

> Demonstration of skilled care requires documentation of the type and level of skilled assistance given to the patient/client, clinical decision making (PT) or problem solving (PTA), and continued analysis of patient progress. This can be expressed by recording both the type and amount of manual, visual, and/or verbal cues used by the therapist to assist the patient/client in completing the exercise/activity completely and correctly.

Erickson ML, McKnight R. *Documentation Basics for the Physical Therapist Assistant, Third Edition* (pp. 87-100)

Objective data used to describe the patient's response to interventions is obtained through various methods and techniques, such as range of motion (ROM) measurements, gross muscle testing, sensation testing, girth measurements, and functional tests. When possible, these methods are based on clearly defined procedures and are therefore reproducible. Using reproducible methods helps to improve the validity and reliability of the data obtained. Because objective data are gathered through reproducible procedures, the information is verifiable and therefore useful for validating the need for physical therapy services. Measurements documented in an interim note are compared with those documented in the initial evaluation and future documentation to demonstrate the patient's progress throughout the episode of care. Objective data help to form a detailed picture of the patient and the problem(s) and are used to guide the physical therapy decision-making process.

It is important to remember that the primary goal of physical therapy should be to impact the individual at the activity or participation level. Documentation of objective data should therefore indicate the patient's functional status. When documenting measurements of body structure and function impairments, it is important to correlate those impairments with limitations in the patient's functional activities. For example, instead of just documenting a limitation in shoulder ROM (right shoulder flexion active range of motion [AROM] 0-110°), you should document how the restriction impacts the individual's daily function (patient right shoulder AROM 0°-110° limiting ability to perform daily tasks including reaching items in kitchen cabinets). Reimbursement is typically tied to improvement in function, thus, the documentation of limitations in a patient's functional abilities helps to justify the need for physical therapy services. Finally, a focus on function helps to motivate patients to participate in interventions because functional activities are more meaningful to them. For example, a patient is not as interested in how many degrees of motion she has available in her shoulder joint, but she is interested in having adequate range so that she can comb her hair.

Interim Note

Objective data found in the interim note should show clear connections with the physical therapist evaluation. Interventions provided by the physical therapist assistant should be included in the plan of care (plan section of a SOAP note), and test and measures documented should demonstrate connections between measurements found in the evaluation and should correlate with goals that are being addressed.

Objective information in an interim note falls into one of the following 3 categories: (1) information that demonstrates the patient's readiness to participate with physical therapy, (2) physical therapy intervention(s) provided, or (3) information that demonstrates the patient's response to the physical therapy intervention provided. Let's take a closer look at these 3 areas and the type of information that you will need to record in an interim note.

Data Indicating That It Is Safe for Patient to Participate in Selected Interventions

Prior to initiating any intervention, you will verify that the patient's physiologic status is adequate for the patient to participate in the activities as planned. Various objective data may need to be evaluated depending upon the patient's condition and the specific intervention(s) provided. For example, you are working with a patient who has had a stroke and is receiving therapy for functional training, including transfers and gait training. Prior to beginning these activities, you would need to ensure that the patient is physiologically safe to participate through assessing the patient's cardiovascular status and general cognitive status. In another example, when working with a patient who is receiving physical therapy for gait training following a total hip replacement, you will want to observe the patient's surgical leg to monitor for symptoms of a deep vein thrombosis. Potential areas and types of data that may need to be performed prior to the initiation of interventions to ensure that the patient is safe to participate include the following [2,3]:

- **Aerobic capacity/endurance:** Heart rate, blood pressure, respiratory rate, and monitor response to position changes (orthostatic hypotension).
- **Balance:** General observation of sitting and/or standing balance.
- **Circulation:** Peripheral pulses, general observations of edema, skin color, and nail color.
- **Mental functions:** Orientation (to situation, time, place, and person), ability to process commands, and level of arousal.
- **Pain:** Location, intensity, and changes with posture/movement.
- **Sensory integrity:** General observations of the patient's ability to process sensory information.
- **Ventilation and respiration:** Oxygen saturation, respiratory rate and rhythm, and skin color.

Interventions Provided

As noted previously, when documenting interventions provided, it is important to include details and to focus on the patient's function. General areas that should be included when documenting interventions area communication and coordination, patient-related instruction, and procedural interventions. Some examples are provided here. Later in the chapter, we look at specific components that need to be included for different interventions.

- **Communication and coordination:** Discussion with the nursing staff about the patient's pain medication schedule.
- **Patient-related instruction:** Education related to hip precautions with a patient who is recovering from a total hip arthroplasty.
- **Procedural interventions:** Transfer and gait training, therapeutic exercise program, and physical agents.

Patient's Response to Physical Therapy Intervention Provided

Documentation of the patient's response to the interventions is essential to demonstrating the patient's progress and to demonstrate that the interventions require the problem-solving skills of a physical therapist assistant. In addition, a full description of interventions provided helps to support billing or timed procedures. Patient's responses can be demonstrated through the following examples:

- **Results of data collected:** Through techniques such as goniometry or manual muscle testing.
- **Description of patient's function:** Description of the patient's ability to move around in bed.
- **Observations about patient:** Any general observations that cannot be categorized as data from a specific technique or a description of function, including information such as description of an open wound, description of patient's movement strategies, or documentation of tenderness to palpation.

Structure/Organization of Objective Section (O)

There is no universal standard structure for the documentation of objective data. Many facilities establish standards that should be followed. In the case where a standard does not exist, the information should be presented in a logical sequence to assist the clinical decision making of all involved in patient care and to allow reviewers of the documentation to determine details about the care provided. To allow for easy identification of data, it is necessary to organize the information with the use of subheadings. You should refer to the initial evaluation and use the same subheadings found there, when possible. This will allow individuals to find information quickly and easily, to correlate the information with the initial evaluation and to determine the patient's progress toward the established goals. In addition, when documenting interventions, it is important to clearly distinguish the intervention from the tests and measures data. This can be accomplished by separating tests and measures data from the interventions data and by clearly labeling each. When you have information that does not easily fall within the subheadings noted in the initial evaluation note, you may choose alternative subheadings. Appropriate subheadings for tests and measures data can be found in Sidebar 2-2. A thorough description of each of area, including definitions, examples of clinical indications, examples of what tests and measures may characterize or quantify, examples of data-gathering tools, and examples of data used in documentation can be found in the APTA *Guide to Physical Therapist Practice.*[2]

In addition to the tests and measures data, you should include an "interventions provided" section. Information in this section should include any collaboration and communication with other health care providers or the physical therapist, patient/client instruction, and all procedural interventions provided.

Often, information in the objective section is best communicated in list, column, or table format. These formats are used to make the information easier to follow. Columns or tables are also used to document comparative data, such as previous status compared with current status or preintervention measurements compared with postintervention measurements. Information that is frequently documented in this format includes goniometric and manual muscle test results.

Example:

	AROM	PROM	Strength
(R) hip abduction	20	30	2-/5
Adduction	0	10	2-/5
Flexion	80	95	3-/5
Extension	0	5	2+/5
(R) Knee	10-100	5-120	3-/5
(R) Ankle DF	5	20	3-/5
PF	45	45	4/5
Inv	20	30	3+/5
Ev	5	15	3+/5

General Tips

- When documenting results of tests and measures, it is important that all pertinent information be included to allow for the reproduction of the test. Standard testing procedures will be assumed, therefore, if any alterations to the procedure are used, they should be clearly detailed.
- Document results of tests and measures in the same manner as they were performed and documented in the physical therapist's initial evaluation note. Use the same scale used in the initial evaluation.

Example 9-1

O: AROM	(L) knee	Pretreatment	Post-treatment
	Flex	0° to 135°	0° to 140°

Strength: (L) LE quads 3+/5, hamstrings 4-/5, mild discomfort noticed with knee extension.

Gait: Able to ambulate 250′ without assistive device or immobilizer independently but does display decreased cadence and guarding. Demonstrates abnormal heel to toe gait pattern and has a tendency to keep LE extended when walking.

Treatment: (L) LE ham curls prone 2 x 10, 5# long are quads 2 x 10 1#, straight leg raise 2 x 10 no weight. Initiated closed chain knee bilateral bends for proprioceptive retraining 3 x 30.

- All data should be recorded in relation to what the patient did, not what the physical therapist assistant did. For example, when documenting gait, the note would read as follows:
    - Gait: Patient ambulated 100' with a straight cane on level surfaces requiring moderate assistance of 1.

      Not
    - Gait: The physical therapist assistant walked the patient 100' providing moderate assistance.
- As with subjective data, complete sentences are not a requirement, as in the above example; however, all pertinent information needs to be included.
- Not all information addressed in the initial evaluation needs to be addressed in each interim note.
    - Only address data obtained while reassessing the patient during the treatment session.
    - It is not necessary to address areas that were found to be within normal parameters in the initial examination/evaluation if those areas are still normal.
- A copy of any written instructions provided to the patient should be included in the medical record and referred to in the objective section of the note.
- Use verbs such as demonstrated, performed, and is.

Tips for Documenting Interventions Provided

When documenting interventions provided, include all information that is necessary to reproduce the activity (Example 9-1), as follows:

- **Intervention provided:** Specify what intervention was provided (eg, modality, exercise, gait training).
- **Intervention amount:** Indicate the dosage or amount of the intervention provided (eg, number of repetitions, distance covered).
- **Equipment used:** Indicate any equipment used during the intervention (eg, transcutaneous electrictrical nerve stimulation, 5-lb weight, standard walker).
- **Parameters:** Provide the parameters/settings used with the equipment (eg, ramp on/off time with electrical modalities, pounds of traction).
- **Treatment area:** Indicate the specific area of the patient's body that was treated (eg, left biceps, insertion of the right deltoid).
- **Patient positioning:** Specify patient positioning used during the session unless it is a standard position for the specific intervention (eg, indicate patient in side lying or indicate exercises were provided in a gravity-reduced position).
- **Details:** Include the duration, frequency, and number and length of rest breaks.
- **Alterations:** Include anything that would not be considered standard practice.
- **Time:** Include the time of each intervention and total treatment time.

In addition, you will want to document the following information related to each of these areas.

Documenting Communication/Coordination

- Any communication with the supervising physical therapist
- Communication with other health care practitioner (eg, physician, registered nurse, occupational therapist, prosthetist)
- Conversations with administrators or case managers
- Phone conversations with any of the above

Documenting Patient-Related Instruction

- Therapeutic activity instruction (eg, home exercise program)
- Precautions/restricted activity (eg, total hip precautions, lifting restrictions)
- Education related to disease process (eg, what is a stroke?)
- Education related to physical therapy procedures (eg, what is ultrasound, and why is it used?)
- Family/caregiver instruction

Procedural Interventions

Procedural interventions are the techniques and procedures used in physical therapy to affect positive change in the patient's condition. The following is a list of categories of interventions. Each is followed by a list of types for each category and some have additional documentation tips.

- Airway clearance techniques
    - Types
        - Breathing strategies (eg, paced breathing, pursed lip breathing)
        - Coughing techniques
        - Secretion mobilization (eg, chest percussion, postural drainage)
- Application of devices and equipment
    - Types
        - Aids for locomotion (eg, crutches, canes, walkers, rollators, manual wheelchairs, power wheelchairs, power-operated vehicles)
        - Orthoses (eg, ankle-foot orthoses, knee-ankle-foot orthoses, body jackets, wrist cock-up splints, shoe inserts)
        - Prostheses
        - Seating and positioning technologies
        - Other assistive technologies to improve safety, function, and independence (eg, transfer boards, mechanical lifts/hoists)
- Biophysical agents
    - Types
        - Biofeedback
        - Compression therapies (eg, compression garments, vasopneumatic compression devices)
        - Cryotherapy (eg, cold packs, ice massage)
        - Electrical stimulation (eg, muscle, nerve)
        - Hydrotherapy (eg, contrast bath, pools, whirlpool tanks)
        - Light agents (eg, laser)
        - Mechanical devices (eg, continuous passive motion device, tilt table, traction devices)
        - Sound agents (eg, ultrasound)
        - Thermotherapy (eg, hot packs, paraffin baths)
    - Information to include in documentation
        - Specific physical or mechanical agent used
        - Patient position
        - Specific area treated
        - Exact settings used
        - Duration of treatment
- Functional training in self-care and domestic, work, community, social, and civic life
    - Types
        - Activities of daily living training (eg, bed mobility, transfer training)
        - Barrier accommodations or modifications
        - Developmental activities
        - Functional training programs (eg, simulated environments and tasks, work conditioning)
        - Instrumental activities of daily living training (eg, school and play activities training)
    - Information to include in documentation
        - Specific activity (eg, bed to wheelchair transfers)
        - Assistive/adaptive devices used
- Integumentary repair and protection techniques (wound management)
    - Types
        - Biophysical agents (eg, electrical stimulation)
        - Debridement (eg, autolytic, mechanical, pulsed lavage with suction)
        - Dressings (including application and removal)
        - Isolation and sterile technique
        - Topical agents
    - Include in documentation
        - Isolation or sterile techniques used (eg, gown, gloves)
        - Type and amount of dressing used
        - Precautions for dressing removal
- Manual therapy techniques
    - Types
        - Manual lymphatic drainage
        - Manual traction
        - Massage
        - Passive ROM
    - Include in documentation
        - Side(s) (right or left), joint(s), and motion(s)
        - Number of repetitions or time
        - Location
        - Type of massage

- Motor function training
  - Types
    - Balance training (eg, developmental activities, motor control training, neuromuscular re-education)
    - Gait and locomotion training (eg, developmental activities, use of assistive devices, wheelchair propulsion)
    - Posture training (postural awareness, postural stabilization activities)
- Therapeutic exercise
  - Types
    - Aerobic capacity/endurance conditioning or reconditioning (eg, movement efficiency, energy conservation training, walking, and wheelchair propulsion programs)
    - Flexibility exercises (eg, ROM, stretching)
    - Neuromotor development training (eg, developmental activities training)
    - Relaxation (eg, breathing strategies, relaxation techniques)
    - Strength, power, and endurance training (eg, active-assistive, active and resistive exercises and task-specific performance training)
  - Include in documentation
    - Specific activities/exercises performed
    - Equipment used
    - Patient position (if not clear by use of equipment)
    - Repetitions
    - Time spent

Response to Interventions

Documentation of the patient's response to interventions will depend somewhat on the type of response and the intervention. Some responses will be recorded in the tests and measures section of the note. Examples include recording pre- and postheart rate and blood pressure readings and documentation of the amount and type of assistance required during gait training. At other times, the patient's response to interventions is embedded in the description of the intervention or immediately follows the description. For example, when documenting the patient's response to shoulder exercises, after a detailed description of the exercise (movement, resistance, etc), you would document the patient difficulty performing the exercise without undesirable substitutions.

Tips for Documenting Results of Data Collected

When documenting results of data collection, include all information needed for the test to be reproduced and for the results to be clearly understood. Be sure to include the following:

- Procedure utilized (eg, goniometry, manual muscle testing, observation)
- Exactly what was measured (eg, right elbow flexion PROM)
- The patient's position

Types of Data Collected

Vital Signs (indicate before and/or after exercise/activity as appropriate)

- Heart rate
  - Location
  - Quality
  - Rate
- Respiratory rate
  - Rate
  - Rhythm
  - Depth
  - Regularity of pattern
- Blood pressure
  - Location, side
  - Systolic over diastolic (eg BP: (R) brachial 120/80)

Anthropometric Characteristics

- Height
- Weight
- Length
- Girth

Muscle Strength

- The measurement range (eg, when documenting strength for right elbow flexors document 3/5 instead of 3)
- What is measured
  - Muscle group (eg, hip flexors)
  - Specific muscles (eg, gluteus maximus)
  - Arrange logically (group per anatomical location [eg, group shoulder musculature together: shoulder flexors 4/5, extensors 4-/5, abduction 4-/5, adduction 4+/5])
  - Use tables or columns to show (B) measurements or before/after measurements

- Any deviation from standard position/protocol (eg, tested hip extension in sidelying due to patient unable to get in prone because of obesity)

Pain

- Results from written pain questionnaires, scales, and diagrams (eg, the McGill Pain Questionnaire, Pain Disability Index, visual analogue scales, pain drawings, pain maps)
- Note: Verbal descriptions of pain given by the patient are often included in the subjective portion of the note. Sometimes, data from pain questionnaires are also recorded in the subjective portion of the interim note.
- Describe patient's nonverbal pain responses to activities, positioning, and postures

Range of Motion

- Document the range from the beginning of the range available to the end of the range available (eg, elbow flexion 5° to 110° instead of just elbow flexion 110°)
- Specific joint
- Arrange logically
- Group per anatomical location
- Use tables or columns to show (B) measurements or before/after measurements
- Any deviation from standard position/protocol (eg, shoulder external rotation; unable to achieve standard test position due to pain restrictions; pt. placed in 45° of abduction for measurement)

Results of Any Standard Tests or Questionnaires

- Record measurements per the standard of the test being used (eg, Berg Balance Scale)

Assistive, Adaptive, Orthotic, Protective, Supportive, and Prosthetic Devices

- Specify device being used (eg, left custom ankle-foot orthosis)
- Discuss patient's (patient's family's/caregiver's) ability to care for device
- Discuss patient's ability to don/doff device as appropriate
- Discuss skin condition related to use of the device
- Discuss safety risks associated with use of the device

Gait, Locomotion, and Balance

- Indicate activity (eg, gait, wheelchair mobility)
- Indicate any assistive, adaptive, orthotic, protective, supportive, or prosthetic devices used (eg, wheeled walker)
- Indicate type of surface the patient is traversing (eg, level surface, stairs)
- Indicate distance traveled or amount of time activity is tolerated (eg, 100 feet, 10 minutes)
- List amount and type of physical assistance provided (eg, patient required minimal assistance to place left lower extremity)
- Number of people needed to aid (eg, patient required minimal assistance of 2 people). If no number is providing, then assume it is 1 person
- List amount and type of cues given (eg, patient required constant verbal cues for cane placement)
- Describe gait pattern used, if appropriate (eg, 4-point gait pattern)
- Describe gait deviations, if appropriate (eg, patient demonstrated left foot drop during swing phase of gait)
- When documenting gait, include weightbearing status

Self-Care, Home Management, and Community or Work Reintegration

- Record measurements of physical environments
- Record any safety concerns or barriers in home, community, and work environments

Results of Any Standard Tests or Questionnaires

- Record measurements per the standard of the test being used (eg, Functional Independence Measure [FIM], 36-Item Short Form Health Survey)

To provide greater objectivity and reliability when documenting functional status, some clinics and facilities use standardized tests or questionnaires to measure impairments, function, and degree of disability. Each test or questionnaire will have specific directions related to appropriate documentation to allow for consistency of administration and scoring. When using a standardized tool, the clinician and facility will want to verify its validity and reliability. Specific tools are designed for specific patient populations. A tool that has been determined to be valid in one setting may not be appropriate in another. Finally, traditional grading of function (eg, independent, minimal assistance) should be consistent with scoring given on standardized instruments. Table 9-1 demonstrates a comparison of documentation of functional status utilizing traditional terminology and scoring utilizing the FIM, a standardized test for measuring a patient's function. Other functional measures can be found in Table 9-2 and in the Rehabilitation Measures Database at www.rehabmeasures.org. The APTA provides its members with an online resource, PTNow, which provides information about many standardized tests. The website provides a description of the test, information about the validity and reliability of the test, a copy of the test, and reference: http://www.ptnow.org/Default.aspx.

Table 9-1

Documentation of Functional Status Using Traditional Terminology Versus FIM Scores

Abbreviation	Definition	Amount/Type of Assistance Needed	FIM Score	Descriptor	Amount/Type of Assistance Needed
(I)	Independent	No assistance needed	7	Complete independence	All of the tasks described as making up the activity are typically performed safely, without modification, assistive devices, or aids, and within a reasonable amount of time
No direct correlation with FIM score			6	Modified independence	One or more of the following may be true: • The activity requires an assistive device • The activity takes more than reasonable time • There are safety risks
SBA	Standby assist	Patient needs someone close by for safety or to provide verbal or visual cues	5	Supervision or setup	Patient requires no more help than standby, cueing or coaxing, without physical contact, or helper sets up needed items or applies orthoses or assistive/adaptive devices
CGA	Contact guard assist	Patient needs someone touching him/her for safety or to provide physical cues	No direct correlation with FIM scores		
Min	Minimal	Patient performs 75% or more of the effort	4	Minimal contact assistance	Patient requires no more help than touching and expends 75% or more of the effort
Mod	Moderate	Patient performs 25% to 75% of the effort	3	Moderate assistance	Patient requires more help than touching or expends half or more of the effort (50% to 75%)
Max	Maximal	Patient performs 25% or less of the activity	2	Maximal assistance	Patient expends less than 50% of the effort but at least 25%

Abbreviations: CGA, contact guard assist; FIM, Functional Independence Measure; (I), independent; Max, maximal; Min, minimal; Mod, moderate; SBA, standby assist.

Table 9-2

Outcome Measures and Their Target Patient Population

Outcome Measure	Patient Population
Acute Care Index of Function (ACIF)	Acute neurological
Arthritis Impact Measurement Scale (AIMS2)	Arthritis
Asthma Quality of Life Questionnaires	Asthma
Cardiac Health Profile	Cardiovascular disease
Dallas Pain Questionnaire	Chronic spinal pain
Diabetes Impact Measurement Scale (DIMS)	Type 1 and type 2 diabetes
Disability Rating Scale	Severe head trauma
Fatigue Impact Scale	Chronic disease
Fibromyalgia Impact Questionnaire	Fibromyalgia
Foot Function Index	Foot pain
Frail Elderly Functional Assessment	Frail elderly
Functional Independence Measure (FIM)	Variety
Functional Performance Inventory	Moderate to severe chronic obstructive pulmonary disease
Fugl-Meyer Assessment Scale	Cerebrovascular accident
Gross Motor Performance Measure (GMPM)	Children with cerebral palsy
Gross Motor Function Measure (GMFM)	Pediatric
Harris Hip Scale	Hip arthritis
Neck Disability Index (NDI)	Neck disorders
Oswestry Low Back Pain Disability Questionnaire	Low back disorders
Parkinson's Disease Quality of Life (PDQL)	Parkinson's disease
Patient-Rated Wrist Evaluation (PRWE)	Wrist disorders
Peabody Development Motor Scales	Pediatric motor development
Pediatric Evaluation of Disability Index (PEDI)	Pediatric
Physical Disability Index	Frail elderly
12-Item Short Form Health Survey (SF-12)	Variety
36-Item Short Form Health Survey (SF-36)	Variety
Sickness Impact Profile (SIP)	Variety with versions for nursing home residents and stroke
Stroke Impact Scale	Cerebrovascular accident
Therapeutic Associates Outcomes System	Variety of musculoskeletal disorders
Western Ontario and McMaster Universitites Osteoarthritis Index	Osteoarthritis
WeeFIM	Pediatric function

Arousal, Mentation, and Cognition

- Describe changes in patient's state of arousal, mentation, and cognition (eg, pt. lethargic today; difficult to arouse and attend to therapeutic activities)

Integumentary Integrity

- Location of wound/skin condition
- Size of wound
- Depth of wound
- Location and depth of any tunneling/undermining
- Description of tissue
- Description of surrounding area
- Description of drainage
- Description of odor
- Activities, positioning, and postures that aggravate or relieve pain, alter sensation, or produce associated skin trauma

Joint Integrity and Mobility

- Describe abnormal joint movements/end feels

Muscle Performance

- Describe abnormal muscle mass (eg, left lower-extremity gastrocnemius atrophy compared to right lower extremity)
- Describe change in muscle tone (eg, noted hypertonicity of right lower extremity during gait with straight cane)

Neuromotor Development

- Describe gross and fine motor milestones
- Describe abnormal righting and equilibrium reactions

Posture

- Describe alignment of trunk
- Describe alignment of extremities in relation to trunk

Ventilation, Respiration, and Circulation Examination

- Describe skin color in relation to circulation and ventilation
- Describe symptoms of ventilation/respiratory or circulatory deficiency
- Describe chest wall expansion and excursion
- Describe cough
- Describe sputum color and consistency

References

1. American Physical Therapy Association. *Defensible documentation for patient/client management.* APTA website. http://www.apta.org/Documentation/DefensibleDocumentation/. Accessed July 13, 2017.
2. American Physical Therapy Association. *Guide to Physical Therapist Practice.* Alexandria, VA: American Physical Therapy Association; 2001. guidetoptpractice.apta.org. Accessed July 13, 2017.
3. American Physical Therapy Association. *Minimum Required Skills of Physical Therapist Assistant Graduates at Entry-Level.* BOD G11-08-09-18. https://www.apta.org/uploadedFiles/APTAorg/About_Us/Policies/BOD/Education/MinReqSkillsPTAGrad.pdf. Updated December 14, 2009. Accessed July 13, 2017.
4. American Physical Therapy Association. *PTnow.* APTA webiste. http://www.ptnow.org/Default.aspx. Accessed July 13, 2017.

Review Questions

1. Describe the type(s) of information that should be documented in the objective portion of a SOAP note.

2. Define reliability and validity.

3. How are data from tests and measures used by the physical therapist assistant to make decisions about provision of selected interventions? How can limitations of objective data be minimized and controlled?

4. When is it important for the physical therapist assistant to document data indicating that body structures and functions or activities are within normal limits?

5. When can tables or columns be used to document objective information? What are the benefits of structuring the information in this format?

Application Exercises

I. Review the list of categories for tests and measures in *Guide to Physical Therapist Practice*. Choose one category from tests and measures (ie, aerobic capacity and endurance), and identify one specific test/measure that can be used to collect data for that category. Identify the tools and procedures used for the test. Research the reliability and validity of that test. Indicate whether the test measures an impairment or function (ie, disability, activity limitation, participation restriction).

II. Write the following statements in a more clear and concise manner, as it would appear in the medical record:

1. The child walked from the classroom to the cafeteria (~500') with the physical therapist assistant providing ~25% assistance using Lofstrand crutches. She required cues at the trunk for rotation and upper and lower body dissociation. She used a 4-point gait pattern. Her lower extremities were externally rotated and knees were in a valgus position. Her hips were adducted.

2. The patient was able to walk in the hallway at the hospital with supervision and no assistive device. Her velocity was 0.8 m/sec.

3. The patient demonstrated the following ROM measurements: passive ROM for right shoulder flexion was 115° and for shoulder extension 10°.

4. The patient propelled his wheelchair down the hallway, onto the elevator, and up and down the ramp in the front of the school. The total distance was ~1000 feet. He required 2 rest breaks for ~2 minutes each. He needed minimal assist to ascend the ramp and turn the wheelchair on the elevator.

5. Prior to initiating interventions, the measurements taken for the cardiovascular system were blood pressure at 135 mm Hg systolic and 90 mm Hg diastolic, heart rate at 98 beats per minute, the patient's oxygen saturation was 98%, and his respiratory rate was 12 breaths per minute.

III. Organize the following information so that it is clear, concise, and suitable for entry into the medical record:

1. The patient's AROM is as follows: Right knee flexion 100°, right knee extension 5°, right hip abduction 20°, right hip flexion 100°, right ankle plantar flexion 20°, left elbow 10°–100°, left shoulder flexion 100°, left shoulder abduction 100°, right hip internal rotation 20°, right ankle dorsiflexion 5°, left shoulder external rotation 60°, left shoulder internal rotation 45°, left hip abduction 25°, left hip extension 0°, right hip extension 5°, right elbow flexion 120°, right elbow extension 0°, right shoulder flexion 165°, left knee flexion 120°, left hip flexion 120°, left hip internal rotation 20°, left hip external rotation 40°, right hip external rotation 45°, left knee extension 0°, left plantar flexion 45°, left dorsiflexion 20°, right shoulder abduction 140°, right shoulder external rotation 80°, and right shoulder internal rotation 45°.

2. You are working with an 8-month-old child with hypotonia and developmental delay. She was able to maintain prone on elbows for 2 minutes independently while given a visual cue. She was able to prop sit with supervision for 30 seconds. The infant was also able to demonstrate a righting reaction to the right but not to the left.

3. The patient with cervical radiculopathy had the following neck AROM measurements: cervical flexion 30° with pain, extension 20°, right lateral flexion 30°, left lateral flexion 25°. His treatment included moist heat for 15 minutes, soft tissue massage for 10 minutes, and 20 repetitions each chin tucks and scapular retractions. He was educated on lifting mechanics and postural correction. He also received intermittent mechanical traction with 15 pounds of pressure with 30 seconds on and 10 seconds off for 10 minutes.

4. The patient with right hemiplegia was able to ambulate 50' twice with a large-based quad cane. She required minimal assist for guarding at her trunk but moderate to maximum assist for achieving full swing, placing the right foot, and stabilizing the right knee during midstance.

5. Wound assessment revealed the following information: The skin around the wound is red, warm to the touch, shiny, and swollen. The wound is a 4 cm × 2.4 cm oval-shaped wound on the dorsum of the foot. It is 1.5-cm deep. The patient has diminished sensation to light touch when compared bilateral. She is unable to feel the 10 g monofilament on the plantar surface of the right foot. Girth at the right metatarsophalangeal joints is 22 cm and 18 cm on the left. The right dorsal pedal pulse is present but diminished compared to the (L), which is 2+.

IV. Review the objective portion of a SOAP note as found in Example 9-1. Critique the note by answering the following questions:

1. Is the information structured logically?

2. Is the information presented in a way that allows for ease of finding pertinent information?

3. Does the objective information provide data that address impairment and function?

4. Does the objective information provide data about the patient's activity limitations or participation restrictions?

5. Does the objective information provide data about the patient's overall disabilities?

V. While working with a patient in a skilled nursing facility who is recovering from a left total hip arthroplasty, the following information is obtained. Organize and write the information so that it is clear, concise, and suitable for entry as an interim note.

Prior to initiating interventions, the following data were gathered: The blood pressure reading was 130/85 mm Hg, heart rate was 88 beats per minute and respiratory rate was 20 breaths per minute. There was a scar that appeared to be healing well on the left hip, surgical staples were present and intact, and there was no drainage from the wound. The following data were gathered during or after the interventions: The patient's left knee musculature measured at a 4+ out of 5 and the ankle musculature measured 5 out of 5. The assistant helped the patient walk in the hallway. The patient was able to walk 50 feet while the assistant provided about 25% assistance. The patient used a standard walker. The assistant provided verbal instructions for sequencing and encouragement to put as much weight as the patient felt comfortable with through the leg. The patient also occasionally placed the walker too far in front of her and the therapist had to remind the patient of the proper walker placement. When the assistant helped the patient up from the bed, the patient needed 25% assistance to scoot over in bed. The assistant primarily helped by moving the operative limb. When sitting on the side of the bed, the patient required more assistance and was able to perform about 50% of the activity. When moving from sitting on the edge of the bed to standing with the walker, the patient performed about 50% of the task.

Chapter 10

Writing the Assessment and Plan Sections

Rebecca McKnight, PT, MS

KEY TERMS Assessment data | Documentation | Evaluation note | Interim note | Plan data | Reimbursement | SOAP note

KEY ABBREVIATIONS PT | PTA | SOAP

Chapter Objectives

After reading this chapter, the reader will be able to do the following:

1. List the type of information that should be recorded in the assessment portion of a SOAP (subjective, objective, assessment, and plan) note.
2. List the type of information that should be recorded in the plan portion of a SOAP note.
3. Describe the importance of the assessment and plan portions of a SOAP note in relationship to reimbursement.
4. Organize given information into a logically structured and well-written assessment portion of a SOAP note.
5. Organize given information into a logically structured and well-written plan portion of a SOAP note.
6. Describe the importance of linking assessment and plan information in the interim note with information in the evaluation note.
7. Organize given information into a complete, logically structured SOAP note following basic documentation guidelines.

The assessment section of the interim SOAP note answers the question, "What does it all mean?" This provides the physical therapist or physical therapist assistant with the opportunity to explain the relevance of the documented data. The assessment is often the most difficult section of the note to write, but is the most important. A key point to remember about writing the assessment is to provide a picture of why skilled services are needed. This is the physical therapist's or the physical therapist assistant's (where allowed by law) opportunity to summarize the patient's progress (or lack thereof), status toward goals, changes in condition, and ongoing impairments, activity limitations, and participation restrictions. This is the place to make obvious how interventions have led to changes in the patient's status. When writing the assessment, it is helpful to imagine that you are talking with an insurance company and you really want to portray the patient's status clearly to ensure that he or she receives appropriate coverage.

The assessment section provides a summary of the subjective and objective information. In this section, you should also include an explanation of how the data demonstrate the patient's response to the intervention(s) provided

Erickson ML, McKnight R. *Documentation Basics for the Physical Therapist Assistant, Third Edition* (pp. 101-109)

and a statement about how the patient is progressing with the goals established in the initial plan of care.

Importance of Documenting the Assessment (A)

As stated in Chapter 3, appropriate documentation is required to meet ethical and legal standards and to communicate with reimbursement bodies such as Medicare & Medicaid. It is within the assessment section of the SOAP note that the physical therapist or the physical therapist assistant documents the patient's need for physical therapy services by showing how the recommended plan of care requires the skills and clinical decision-making/problem-solving abilities of a physical therapist or a physical therapist assistant.

When applicable, you should indicate how interventions have led to changes in the patient's status. Information in the assessment section should clearly describe the patient's response to the intervention(s) provided and the patient's progress in reference to the goals established in the plan of care/initial evaluation. This information should clearly demonstrate why continuation of skilled services is needed. You need to be concise but also specific. General phrases such as, "The patient tolerated the treatment well" or "The patient is progressing toward stated goals" should be avoided. These phrases do not delineate the skill or decision-making requirements necessary to justify physical therapy.[1]

Explanation of How Data Demonstrate Patient's Response to Intervention

To demonstrate the need for skilled services, it is important to explain the connection between the tests and measure information found in the objective section and the interventions provided. All references to improvements in impairments (eg, range of motion, strength) should be correlated with functional tasks. Examples include the following:

- **Change in patient's pain level.** For example, you are providing transcutaneous electrical nerve stimulation application for pain control for a patient with chronic back pain with radicular symptoms. Prior to initiating intervention, the patient rates his pain as 7/10. The patient rates his pain as 2/10 after initiation of transcutaneous electrical nerve stimulation trial. In the assessment component of the note, you can highlight the significant reduction in patient reports of pain after implementation of the electrotherapeutic intervention. It is also important to relate the change in pain rating with a functional task. For example, in the scenario above, perhaps prior to the intervention, the patient was unable to bend down to remove his shoes. After the application, however, he was able to easily don/doff his shoes.
- **Change in patient's impairment**. For example, you are assisting with the care of a patient who has lymphedema. You are using volumetric measurements to document the amount of edema before and after intervention. In the assessment section, you do not need to restate the measurements, as they will be in the objective section of the note, but you should refer to the amount of change and indicate any significant impact on functional abilities. A patient with upper-extremity lymphedema, for instance, may have difficulty grasping objects. After interventions, the patient may be able to pick up a pencil.
- **Changes in patient's functional abilities and ability to participate in larger social settings (eg, work, school).** For example, after a few therapy sessions, the patient might report the ability to perform bathing at home independently when he was unable to do so before.

Patient's Progress Toward Goals

When addressing patient goals in the assessment section of the interim note, you will want to review the initial evaluation and all follow-up documentation related to progression toward goal achievement. In your interim note, you should comment on every goal that has not previously been achieved. For example, an initial evaluation indicated 7 goals. Upon review of follow-up documentation, you note that 2 of those goals have been achieved. In your interim note, you will need to comment on the 5 additional goals that have not yet been achieved. Further, if new or additional goals have been added by the physical therapist assistant during a re-evaluation, you will need to comment on those goals as well. For each goal you are addressing, you will indicate one of the following:

- A goal has been achieved.
- Progress has been made toward a goal.
- No progress has been made toward a goal.
- A decline in patient status as related to a goal has occurred (Example 10-1).

When addressing each goal, you need to reference information from the tests and measures as evidence to support your statement. For example, a goal indicates that a patient will be independent with gait on level surface and up/down stairs using a straight cane. At the initiation of physical therapy, the patient needed minimal assistance for balance constantly, for correct placement of the cane occasionally, for correct placement of the affected lower extremity frequently, and for verbal cues for sequencing frequently. At the time that you are writing an interim note, the patient

Example 10-1

Assessment Component of an Interim Note

A: Showing improvement in ROM and strength and functional gait. ROM has increased from 5 degrees-90 degrees at the initial examination to 0 degrees-140 degrees meeting STG #2 leading to decreased gait deviations. Strength of quads have increased from 2/5 to 3+/5; ham have increased from 3+/5 to 4-/5 meeting short-term goal #3. Will continue to work toward STGs 1 & 4 and all LTGs.

still needs minimal assistance; however, now the assistance is for balance occasionally and for verbal cues for correct placement of cane and affected lower extremity occasionally. Verbal cues are no longer necessary for the sequencing of the gait pattern. The details of the patient's status should be found in the objective section of the note, but it is essential that you highlight the comparison between the patient's status at the time of the initial evaluation compared with his or her current status. Without providing the comparison of the details, it will appear that the patient has not made any progress since the amount of assistance provided in general is still "minimal."

Patient's Continued Need for Physical Therapy Services

Once you have clearly demonstrated the patient's progress, you can then address the continued need for skilled services. You should be able to point to the additional components that need to be addressed. For example, in the previous case, you could state that the patient continues to require physical assistance and verbal cueing and will benefit from additional functional training as outlined in the physical therapist's plan of care. If the patient's status has declined or no progress has been made, it is important for you to draw connections with any event that might be a factor. For example, a patient receiving home health services may have had a stomach illness and therefore demonstrated a decline in performance. You will have documented the patient's report of the stomach illness in the subjective section and can refer to this when pointing out that the patient's status has either not improved or has declined.

Tips for Writing the Assessment (A)

- There should never be any information in the assessment section that does not relate to data documented in the subjective and objective sections.
- Back up all statements with data from the subjective and objective sections. For example, if you document that the patient has an improvement in his or her mobility, refer to the data documented in the objective section that substantiate that comment.
- Be specific. Do not simply document items such as, "Tolerated treatment well" or "Patient progressing." Always indicate how you know these things.[1]
- In keeping with the *International Classification of Functioning, Disability and Health* disablement model,[2] you should indicate relationships between impairments, activity limitations, and participation restrictions in this section. For example, the following statement would be very appropriate:
  "A: Pt. continues to have decreased AROM in the (R) shoulder limiting her ability to dress and reach into her overhead cabinets."
- The effect of the interventions on activity limitations and participation restrictions should be highlighted. The following statement demonstrates this:
  "A: Pt. demonstrating improved ROM in the (R) shoulder since starting HEP. Improvement in ROM has allowed better ability to dress and reach into overhead cabinets."
- Demonstrate the relationship between the current status and goals.

Plan (P)

The final component of a SOAP note is the plan. The plan section of an interim SOAP note answers the question, "Where do we go from here?" The plan should be based on the established plan of care and the patient's response to the interventions and progression toward goals. The plan will delineate what actions need to occur within the following: (1) coordination/communication, (2) patient/client-related instructions, and (3) procedural interventions. Within the plan part of the interim note, you should record what interventions will be provided in upcoming sessions and you should refer to the goals that those interventions are addressing. Specific session objectives should also be noted when appropriate. For example, when working with a patient with several factors impacting functional gait, you may choose to focus on just one parameter for the upcoming session (eg, weight shifting). Your plan can indicate, "Gait training next session will focus on weight shifting to improve balance and to allow for an increased stride length." The types of information that should be in the plan section of an interim note include the following:

- Coordination/communication
  - Request for a re-examination/re-evaluation by the physical therapist (eg, patient is not progressing as desired with the current plan of care/treatment plan).

Example 10-2

Plan Component of Interim Note

P: Continue physical therapy in the outpatient setting 3 x/wk for strengthening, proprioceptive exercises, and gait training. Next session, increase focus on closed chain exercises to improve proprioception. Focus on heel to toe gait activities during gait training.

Jody Laughlin, PTA

- Consultation with the physical therapist (eg, to determine strategies to try to improve the efficacy of the intervention).
- Information that the physical therapist needs to be advised about (eg, patient's plans have changed from returning home alone upon discharge to moving in with a family member).
- Communication with other health care providers (eg, discussing discharge plans with a social worker).

- Patient-/client-related instructions
  - Written instruction to be provided (eg, will issue and instruct in home exercise program [HEP] next session).
  - Education regarding activity restrictions and precautions (eg, will educate patient regarding hip precautions and car transfers).
- Procedural interventions
  - Progression of the treatment plan within the established plan of care (eg, will increase resistance with therapeutic exercises).
  - Modification of the treatment plan within the established plan of care (eg, will change from using a standard walker to using a wheeled walker due to patient's continued problems with appropriate sequencing while using the standard walker).
  - Equipment to be purchased (eg, wheeled walker for home use).
  - Activities to perform (eg, will focus on bed mobility training).
  - Schedule for continued therapy (eg, to continue with twice daily treatments with anticipated discharge in 3 days to home).

Tips for Writing the Plan (P)

- Use phrases such as, "Will check," "Will update," "Will consult," "Will increase," and "Will hold."
- The plan should include anything that you are thinking about doing with the patient.
- Indicate why treatments you are planning are medically necessary (eg, will initiate light strengthening next visit to reduce atrophy and weakness associated with immobilization).
- This should serve as a reminder to you during the patient's next session and provide a guide for the next physical therapist or physical therapist assistant treating the patient (Example 10-2).

Now that you know basic documentation principles and specific guidelines for documenting patient care in a SOAP note format, you should be able to adapt and document this information in an appropriate manner, regardless of the policies and styles that you are presented with in the clinical situations that you encounter.

Pulling It All Together

The American Physical Therapy Association *Guidelines: Physical Therapy Documentation of Patient/Client Management* indicates that "documentation is required for every patient visit/encounter."[3] The primary purposes of a treatment, interim, or daily note is to document what occurred during that session or on that day in relation to the patient's physical therapy services and to support the billing codes that were used. Documentation of the patient visit should include the following elements: (1) subjective reports from the patient; (2) specific interventions provided during the session that are consistent with what was billed; (3) the patient's response to the interventions provided, including objective improvements made; (4) changes in patient impairment, activity limitation, and participation restriction; (5) any equipment or written instruction provided to the patient; (6) any factor leading to a modification of the plan of care; and (7) any communication or collaboration with other health care providers regarding the patient's care.[3] To ease time constraints and facilitate consistency between clinicians, interventions are often documented through the use of standard forms, checklists, flowsheets, or graphs.

Structure of an Interim SOAP Note

The structure and organization of an interim SOAP note will be like the structure and organization of the evaluation note. At the beginning of the note, you will need to provide the patient's name and the date the services were provided. The subjective section includes the patient's remarks regarding his or her condition, the intervention, and the changes in impairment or function brought on by the treatment. When documenting objective data, it is important to clearly differentiate between tests and measures data that have been collected to illustrate the patient's status and interventions that were provided. The latter is frequently accomplished by the utilization of tables or flowsheets for documentation of specific interventions. Alternatively, this can be accomplished by using subheadings (ie, Impairments, Functional Status, Coordination of Care, Patient-Related Instruction, and Procedural Interventions). As noted earlier in this chapter, the assessment section should include information regarding the patient's response to the interventions provided and his or her progress toward the stated goals. It is important to reference both the initial evaluation and the information found in the subjective and objective sections of the interim note to craft the assessment information. The note ends with the physical therapist assistant outlining what activities will occur in the future related to the patient's physical therapy care. Finally, you will need to sign your name. Signing your name is the process known as authentication, defined as "the process used to verify that the entry is complete, accurate and final."[3]

References

1. Clifton DW Jr. "Tolerated treatment well" may no longer be tolerated. *PT Magazine.* 1995;3(10):24.
2. World Health Organization. *International Classification of Functioning, Disability and Health.* Geneva, Switzerland: World Health Organization; 2001. http://apps.who.int/iris/bitstream/10665/42407/1/9241545429.pdf. Accessed July 2, 2017.
3. American Physical Therapy Association. *Guidelines: Physical Therapy Documentation of Patient/Client Management.* BOD G 03-05-16-41. http://www.apta.org/uploadedFiles/APTAorg/About_Us/Policies/Practice/DocumentationPatientClientManagement.pdf. Updated December 14, 2009. Accessed July 7, 2017.

Review Questions

1. What type of information is found within the assessment and plan portions of the SOAP note?

2. How should an interim note be structured? How should the information relate to the initial evaluation?

Application Exercises

I. Write the following information in a clear, concise manner, as it would appear in the medical record.

1. Upon arrival in the outpatient department for her follow-up visit, the patient indicates that she has been doing her HEP without any problems and that she feels that she is able to don her coat, reach for her car door and seat belt, and perform light household chores without difficulty.

2. You have been treating a patient with plantar fasciitis, providing ultrasound, soft tissue massage, and stretching. On the third visit, the patient indicates that his pain in the morning has decreased from 5/10 to 3/10. His active and passive dorsiflexion range of motion have increased 5°. During gait, he has increased his stance time on the involved extremity.

3. The 8-year-old child with spastic diplegia is now able to walk with standby assist from her classroom to the bathroom (~150') with a posterior walker. At the beginning of the school year (3 months ago), she was only able to walk 50' with minimal assist of 1.

4. You are assisting an 18-year-old female patient who injured her knee playing basketball in walking with crutches. The patient walks in the hallway for 100' without your help. When the patient attempts to walk up the stairs, she tells you that it scares her. You must keep a hand on her to provide minimal stability for her to get up and down 1 physical therapist 1 flight of stairs. At the last visit, she could only ascend and descend 3 steps. You are planning to continue with increasing her independence on the stairs. She is not allowed to bear any weight on the injured lower extremity.

5. You are working with a 42-year-old patient who is recovering from spinal meningitis. The patient currently needs moderate assistance to perform transfers to and from the wheelchair with a slideboard. The patient also requires occasional verbal cues for setting up the equipment for the transfer. Last week, the patient required maximum assist for the slideboard transfer. The initial plan of care includes a goal for the patient to be independent. You plan on continuing with slideboard transfers and mobility training twice a day.

II. The following is an initial examination and evaluation for a patient recently admitted to an inpatient rehabilitation hospital. Use it to help you complete the 2 SOAP notes that follow.

Initial Examination and Evaluation

Pr: (L) CVA, (R) hemiparesis

Hx: This 67 y.o. male pt. was admitted to the acute care 08-08-11 due to sudden weakness in his (R) UE and LE and slurred speech. Pt.'s PMH includes NIDDM, CABG x 2 07-05-08. No other pertinent medical history.

S: *c/o:* Inability to move around like he used to. Weakness in (R) LE and UE.
Prior level of function:(I) c all ADLs and gait s assistive device. Active; worked in his woodshop, yard, and garden. Pt. is (R) handed.
Home situation: Lives c wife who is healthy but is a small woman. Lives in 2-level home c 4 steps to enter.

O: *Observation*: Noted 3+ pitting edema in (R) hand and forearm; pt. has tendency to keep (R) UE in dependent position.
Sensation: Pt. displays diminished light touch, deep pressure localization, proprioception and kinesthesia through the (R) UE and LE.
Tone: Pt. displays diminished tone on (R) UE and LE to passive range, diminished patellar reflexes and absent Achilles reflex on (R).

MMT: (L) UE and LE: 5/5 throughout all musculature. (R) UE: shoulder flex, ext, abd, MR & LR 2-/5; elbow flex 2+/5, ext 2/5; grip 1/5; (R) LE: hip ext, add, IR 3+/5; flex, add, LR 2+/5; knee ext 3-/5, flex 2-/5; ankle DF 0/5, PF 1/5.

Mobility: Max (A) scooting up in bed, mod (A) scooting (R) and (L) in bed; SBA for safety and v/c when rolling to (R); max (A) rolling to (L).

Transfers: Supine ↔ sit max (A) x 1 from (R) side and mod (A) x 1 from (L) side; sit to stand max (A) x 1; stand pivot w/c ↔ bed max (A) x 1.

Gait: Not attempted at this time.

Balance: Fair– static and poor dynamic sitting balance; standing balance very poor.

Endurance: Fair; pt. tolerated 30-minute session requiring 1-minute rest breaks every 5-8 minutes.

A: *PT Dx*: Impaired motor function and muscular performance due to CVA. Prognosis is good for goals as stated. Skilled service needed to help patient improve strength and functional mobility including gait and transfers so that he can return home.

Problem List:

- Edema in (R) UE
- Decreased strength (R) UE and LE
- Dependent bed mobility
- Dependent transfers
- Nonambulatory
- Diminished balance
- Diminished endurance

STGs to be met in 2 weeks:

1. Pt. will be able to demonstrate understanding of appropriate positioning for (R) UE.
2. Pt. will demonstrate an increase in strength (R) UE and LE ½ grade throughout to allow improved mobility and use of UE.
3. Pt. will require mod (A) scooting up in bed, min (A) scooting (R) and (L) in bed; mod (A) rolling to (L) and be (I) rolling to (R).
4. Pt. will require mod (A) for supine to sit from (R), min (A) supine to sit from (L), mod (A) for sit ↔ stand and w/c ↔ bed transfers.
5. Pt. will stand c max (A) x 1 and quad cane for 1 minute.
6. Pt. will display fair static and fair– dynamic sitting balance and fair– static standing balance.
7. Pt. will display adequate endurance to tolerate a 30-minute therapy session only needing 1 2-minute rest break.

LTGs to be met in 4 weeks:

1. Pt. will be (I) in (R) UE self-care.
2. Pt. will demonstrate an increase in strength (R) UE and LE 1 grade throughout to allow improved mobility and use of UE.
3. Pt. will be (I) c bed mobility including scooting up and down in bed and rolling to (R) or (L).
4. Pt. will be (I) c sit ↔ stand and w/c ↔ bed transfers.
5. Pt. will ambulate 20' c assistive device as indicated and mod (A) x 1 to allow some household ambulation.
6. Pt. will display good static and dynamic sitting balance, fair+ static and fair dynamic standing balance.
7. Pt. will display adequate endurance for a 1-hour session of therapy only 1 5-minute rest break.

P: PT bid for neuromuscular reeducation, strengthening, mobility training, pregait activities, endurance activities, balance training, and education related to positioning and self-care.

Mary Jane, DPT

1. Today, the patient states that he feels that he is getting stronger and is looking forward to his first day pass to go home with his wife this weekend. The patient's wife states that she is concerned about how they will manage in the long run. She says that their son and daughter-in-law are coming in from out of town to help this weekend. In therapy today, you worked on his bed mobility and transfers. He needed moderate assistance when scooting up and down in bed and scooting to the right. He needed minimal assistance when scooting to the left. He could roll to the right without any assistance and was safe with the activity. He required moderate assistance when rolling to the left. The patient still displays significant edema in his right hand and forearm and forgets to use his positioning devices in bed and in the wheelchair. He required minimal assistance when coming up from his left side. He required minimal assistance when performing a sit-to-stand transfer and moderate assistance with a stand pivot transfer from the therapy mat into the wheelchair. You educated the patient's wife regarding his need for supervision and constant verbal cues to perform wheelchair setup and because he is impulsive and unsafe at times. Review the initial evaluation note so that you can make appropriate comparisons with his initial status. Be sure to include a summary of how he is progressing toward his goals and write an appropriate plan.

2. One week later, the patient has returned from a weekend pass with his family. The family had considerable difficulty caring for the patient at home and they feel that the home is not set up well for caring for him. The patient is upset at how difficult it was to be at home. He needs a lot of extra encouragement today to participate in therapy. During his therapy session today, the patient required moderate to maximal assistance with rolling and scooting in bed and for supine to sit transfers when coming up from his right side, and minimal assistance when coming up from his left side. He required maximal assistance when performing a sit-to-stand transfer and moderate assistance with a modified stand pivot transfer from the therapy mat into the wheelchair. The patient needed moderate assistance and constant verbal cues to perform setup and was impulsive and a safety risk today more so than usual due to his bad mood associated with his weekend. In your note, include a summary of how these findings compare with findings from the previous note and the initial evaluation note. Also, briefly comment on the status of his goals and write an appropriate plan.

Chapter 11

Payment Basics

Mia L. Erickson, PT, EdD, CHT, ATC

KEY TERMS Advance beneficiary notice of noncoverage | Alternative payment model | Case-mix groups | Centers for Medicare & Medicaid Services | Copayment | Current procedural terminology | Deductible | Diagnosis-related group | Durable medical equipment | First-party payment | Functional Independence Measure | Health maintenance organization | Home health resource group | Inpatient prospective payment system | Inpatient rehabilitation facility | Inpatient rehabilitation facility patient assessment instrument | Medicare administrative contractor | Medicare allowable | Medicare Part A | Medicare Part B | Medicare Part C | Medicare Part D | Medicare physician fee schedule | Merit-based incentive payment system | Minimum data set | Outcome and assessment information set | Physician quality reporting system | Point of service plan | Preferred provider organization | Primary care physician | Prospective payment system | Quality payment program | Reimbursement | Resource-based relative value scale | Resource utilization group | Skilled nursing facility | Social Security | Third-party payment

KEY ABBREVIATIONS ABN | APM | CMS | CPT | DRG | FIM | HMO | IPPS | IRF | IRF PAI | MAC | MACRA | MDS | MIPS | MPFS | OASIS | PCP | POS | PPO | PPS | PQRS | RBRVS | RUG | SNF

Chapter Objectives

After reading this chapter, the reader will be able to do the following:

1. Define reimbursement.
2. Differentiate between first- and third-party payers.
3. Differentiate between different types of insurance, such as social, managed care, casualty, and indemnity.
4. Explain the differences between Medicare Parts A, B, C, and D, and Medicaid.
5. Examine Medicare reimbursement in a variety of settings (inpatient hospitals, inpatient rehabilitation hospitals, skilled nursing facilities (SNFs), home health care, and outpatient facilities).
6. Examine strategies for cost containment utilized by managed care organizations.
7. Realize how documentation is tied to reimbursement.
8. Construct a physical therapy progress note using basic principles for maximum reimbursement.

What Is Reimbursement?

There are generally 3 parties involved in the financial management of an individual's medical care, as follows: (1)

Erickson ML, McKnight R. *Documentation Basics for the Physical Therapist Assistant, Third Edition* (pp. 111-117)

the patient (first-party); (2) the health care provider, such as the physician, physical therapist, occupational therapist (second-party); and (3) the insurance company (third-party). When a patient receives a service from a health care provider, some form of payment is expected. This payment can come directly from the patient (first-party payment), but more often it comes from the patient's insurance company. Payment to the health care provider from the insurance company is known as third-party payment or reimbursement. The American Physical Therapy Association has defined reimbursement as payment by the patient (first-party) or insurer (third-party) to the health care provider for services provided.[1] The financial success and viability of physical therapy departments and clinics can be dependent upon payment from patients or third-party payers. In the past, physical therapists were paid, or reimbursed, 100% of what they billed. Today, however, this is not the case. Instead, providers are usually paid a percentage of what is billed. There are also many rules and regulations governing the amount of money paid to providers for their services, and they vary according to different insurance companies, insurance policies and contracts, and payers.

Types of Payment

Physical therapy providers receive payment from different types of insurance companies. A brief description of common payment structures is provided in this chapter.

Social Insurance

Social insurance is a form of economic hazard insurance where payment is controlled by supervised government programs. It is available for individuals of advanced age, people with disabilities, and people who are unemployed. Acceptance into a social insurance program is not guaranteed, and individuals seeking acceptance must meet certain criteria.[2] Examples of social insurance available in the United States are Medicare and Medicaid.

A 1965 Amendment to the Social Security Act established the Medicare program.[3] Today, Medicare provides benefits to the following[4]:

- Individuals 65 years of age or older who are US citizens or permanent legal residents who have lived in the United States for at least 5 years; and the individuals or spouses have worked long enough to be eligible for Social Security or railroad retirement benefits or the individuals or spouses are government employees or retirees who have not paid into Social Security but have paid Medicare payroll tax while working.
- Individuals under 65 years of age who have been entitled to Social Security disability benefits for at least 24 months, have end-stage renal disease, or permanent kidney failure with dialysis or transplant, and the individuals or spouses have paid Social Security taxes for a certain length of time, depending on their age; have Lou Gehrig's disease (amyotrophic lateral sclerosis); or receive a disability pension from the Railroad Retirement Board and meet certain conditions.
- From 1977 to 2001, Medicare and Medicaid services were coordinated under the Health Care Financing Administration (HCFA). In 2001, HCFA changed its name to the Centers for Medicare & Medicaid Services (CMS).[5] CMS is a federal agency housed in the US Department of Health & Human Services. CMS administers the Medicare program and oversees individual state Medicaid programs, such as the Children's Health Insurance Program (CHIP), a program for uninsured children.[6]

Medicare

Medicare is a federally funded program that originally consisted of the following 2 parts: Medicare Part A and Medicare Part B. Medicare Part A covers inpatient hospital stays, SNFs, hospice, and home health services. Medicare beneficiaries (individuals who receive Medicare benefits) typically do not pay a fee for Medicare Part A. This payment came from monthly payroll deductions while the individual or a spouse was employed. Also, enrollment in Part A is automatic for individuals receiving Social Security benefits. Medicare Part B, or Medical Insurance Part B, pays for physician visits and services, laboratory work, diagnostic imaging, outpatient surgeries, preventive services, and medically necessary durable medical equipment such as walkers.[7]

Other parts of Medicare include Parts C and D. Medicare Part C consists of Medicare Advantage Plans. These plans are offered and administered by private insurance companies that are approved by Medicare. Part C includes both Part A and Part B (and, in some instances, Part D) as described above, but each of the Advantage Plans has different costs and coverage. Beneficiaries may choose to enroll in original Medicare (Parts A and B) or Part C. Medicare Part D is Medicare's Prescription Drug Plan and is optional for Medicare beneficiaries.

For Medicare Parts A and B, Medicare contracts with private insurance companies to pay the bills. For Part A and some Part B plans, these companies are known as Medicare Administrative Contractors (MACs).[8] MACs are determined by defined geographic regions.[8] It is important to know the payers for your region so that you can become familiar with their reimbursement and documentation guidelines, as they may differ.

Medicare reimbursement varies depending on the type of facility in which you practice. Different payment systems are in place for different practice settings. Prospective payment systems (PPS) are a type of Medicare reimbursement based on a predetermined, fixed amount.[9] A PPS is in place for acute care hospitals, inpatient rehabilitation hospitals, SNFs, long-term care hospitals, home health care, hospice, hospital outpatient departments, and inpatient psychiatric facilities.[9] Under PPS, the payment amount is derived from patient classification systems specific to the setting (eg, acute care, inpatient rehabilitation). Upon admission to one of these facilities or services, patients are "grouped" according to common characteristics, such as severity of illness or resource consumption. These are known as case-mix groups.[10] For each case-mix group, Medicare has agreed to reimburse the facility a predetermined, fixed amount. The facility's admissions data, or, in some settings, data from standardized evaluation tools, are used to assign patients to a case-mix group.

The PPS in inpatient acute care hospitals is known as the inpatient prospective payment system (IPPS). Under the IPPS, each patient is categorized into a Diagnosis-Related Group (DRG). A DRG is a classification system used to group patients according to diagnosis, type of treatment, age, and other relevant criteria.[10] Hospitals are paid a set, predetermined amount according to the patient's DRG category, regardless of the actual cost to provide care to the patient.[10]

Reimbursement provided to SNFs can occur through Medicare Parts A or B. Payment under Part A is determined through information provided in the case-mix classification system for SNFs known as the resource utilization groups (RUGs) IV. In this system, patients are assigned to a RUG level based on data provided in the resident assessment, the Minimum Data Set 3.0 (MDS 3.0), and the geographic region.[11] The MDS 3.0 is a multidisciplinary assessment performed by a variety of health care providers (eg, physicians, physical therapists, occupational therapists, speech therapists, nurses) that includes data such as status on activities of daily living, hearing, speech, vision, functional status, and cognitive patterns.[12]

Reimbursement to inpatient rehabilitation facilities (IRFs) is similar to that for a SNF, with a few exceptions. Like SNFs, upon admission to an IRF, patients are assessed using an Inpatient Rehabilitation Facility Patient Assessment Instrument (IRF PAI). These data are used to classify patients based on clinical characteristics and anticipated resource needs.[13] Payments are determined based on the patient's classification. However, the Functional Independence Measure (FIM)[14] is the integral part of the IRF PAI for rehabilitation practitioners in these settings. The FIM is administered for all patients in this setting, and the scores are used as data on the IRF PAI.

Patient case-mix groups in home health care are also determined by assessment data collected during the admissions process, similar to SNFs and IRFs; however, in home health, the assessment tool is known as the Outcome and Assessment Information Set (OASIS).[15] Data from the OASIS are used to categorize patients into 1 of 153 Home Health Resource Groups, and payment is predetermined for each group.[16]

Each setting has unique assessment tools and guidelines for reimbursement by Medicare. It is important to point out that, although reimbursement has been predetermined for each of the case-mix groups, payments can be adjusted based on geographic location and cost of providing services to particularly complex patients. Reimbursement can also be adjusted for teaching hospitals and for providers who treat a large number of patients without insurance. It is also important to point out that, in the aforementioned settings, the physical therapist's evaluation informs the multidisciplinary assessment and serves as 1 source of data that establishes the amount that facilities are reimbursed for a particular patient. It is important for the physical therapist to accurately document all comorbidities, complexities, and functional problems so that the patient is accurately categorized.

Reimbursement provided to hospital-based physical therapy outpatient clinics and physical therapy private practices is based on the Medicare Physician Fee Schedule (MPFS).[17] Fee schedules are predetermined lists of payment amounts used by health plans to pay doctors or other providers for various services or procedures performed by physicians or health care providers.[10] This predetermined amount is also known as the Medicare allowable. The MPFS is the PPS for physical, occupational, and speech therapy provided in these settings.

The Medicare allowable is determined by a coding system. First, all health care services or procedures are assigned a 5-digit code under the Current Procedural Terminology (CPT) coding system.[1] This is known as the procedure's CPT code. Under the CPT system, physical therapy procedures generally begin with 97. Each of the CPT codes is then assigned a weight based on the resources it takes to provide. Specifically, payments are determined by the following: (1) the provider work needed to administer the procedure; (2) the practice expense or how much it costs to perform a procedure; and (3) the professional liability insurance (malpractice) value.[18] The professional liability value can be thought of as the associated risk involved with administering a procedure. For example, a joint mobilization has a higher weight than the application of a hot pack or cold pack because a joint mobilization requires more technical skill and has higher associated risk. The scale used for weighting the procedures is known as the resource-based relative value scale (RBRVS).[18] Each CPT code corresponds with an RBRVS value. Once the RBRVS value has been determined, it is multiplied by a conversion factor to establish the Medicare allowable.

After the conversion factor is applied, the dollar value is then adjusted for the geographic region, or practice location, and that becomes the Medicare allowable for the procedure. In addition to Medicare, other third-party payers use the CPT coding system and the RBRVS to establish fee schedules; however, the amount reimbursed by Medicare might vary (higher or lower) from the amount reimbursed by private or nongovernment insurance companies.

Importantly, there are new payment models being explored by Medicare that are based on quality improvement. The Medicare Access and CHIP Reauthorization

Act of 2015 (MACRA) was passed to help in reforming the Medicare payment system, creating a new framework to reward providers for providing high-quality care.[19] According to a new Quality Payment Program established by this legislation, providers will have 2 ways to participate in quality improvement programs, with the first being the Merit-based Incentive Payment System (MIPS) and the second being an advanced Alternative Payment Model (APM).[20] The MIPS program combines 3 existing programs (the Physician Quality Reporting System [PQRS], electronic health record meaningful use, and the value-based system) and then adds a fourth component (improvement activities).[19] An APM shifts payment away from the fee-for-service models that have typically been used. One example of an APM is the Bundled Payments for Care Improvement Initiative where a single, bundled payment is provided to multiple providers who participate in the episode of care.[21]

Prior to 2017, physical therapists in some settings were required to report data from quality measures in the initial examination documentation under the PQRS. However, under the new Quality Payment Program, physical therapists are not required to report MIPS data until 2019.[20]

There are some procedures that are not covered or may not be covered by Medicare. If a health care provider believes that a patient with original Medicare would benefit from a procedure that Medicare probably (or certainly) will not pay for, the provider must have the patient sign an Advance Beneficiary Notice of Noncoverage (ABN).[22] An ABN must be signed on each day that the service is provided. An ABN serves to provide and verify communication to Medicare beneficiaries of their financial responsibility for services that will be or could be denied. An ABN is not required for items or services that Medicare never covers.[22]

Medicaid

Medicaid is a joint federal- and state-funded program that pays for medical care for individuals and families with low incomes.[23] The Affordable Care Act provided states the authority to expand Medicaid eligibility to individuals under age 65 years in families with incomes below 133% of the Federal Poverty Level and standardized the rules for determining eligibility.[23]

Managed Care

Managed care is a type of health care in which the insurance company (payer) contracts with health care providers, including physical therapists, to provide services at a reduced cost to its members. These health care providers make up the plan's network.[24] There are different types of managed care plans, including health maintenance organizations (HMOs), preferred provider organizations (PPOs), and point of service (POS) plans. An HMO plan only pays for care within its network. The patient chooses a primary care physician (PCP) who coordinates the care. A PPO plan also includes a network of providers but, unlike HMOs, PPOs often include out-of-network coverage, although there is usually an increased cost to the patient. A POS plan allows the patient to choose between an HMO and a PPO each time care is needed.[24]

In the past, physical therapy providers could submit a bill and expect to be reimbursed 100% of the amount billed; however, that is not the case today. Managed care insurance contracts are negotiated, and providers often agree to accept a lower amount to be a provider for the particular insurance company or to be included in an insurance company's network. Thus, health care providers accept a reduction in the amount that they are reimbursed. In these plans, there is a predetermined fee schedule, such as the MPFS.

Managed care organizations and many third-party payers use additional strategies to control money paid to providers to contain costs. Any of the following may be used[25]:

- **Using a PCP to control access to specialist care:** At one time, a patient could choose any provider for his or her health care needs. Now, in some managed care plans, the patient's family doctor, or PCP, is the patient's point of access into the health care system. The PCP can then direct the patient's care or refer the patient to a specialist. Under this system, when patients are referred to a specialist through their PCPs, they are provided maximum insurance coverage. However, if they enter the health care system without a PCP referral, their amount of coverage is reduced.
- **Requiring prior authorization:** When prior authorization is required, the provider must contact the insurance company (payer) prior to providing a service and outline the treatment/services that he or she wishes to carry out. The insurance company may or may not give the provider authorization to perform the recommended service. When prior authorization is required, the insurance company does not reimburse services that have not been approved. Payment for orthotic devices, braces, and/or medical equipment used by physical therapists and physical therapist assistants may require prior authorization by some insurance companies.
- **Limiting the number and duration of services provided:** Some insurance companies have policies where there is an established limit on the number of physical therapy visits that will be reimbursed or a time period for which the services will be covered. There can be a lot of variability between insurance companies and between plans within the same company. For example, a patient might be allowed 6 visits per diagnosis or 25 visits per calendar year, regardless of diagnosis. There are also cases where the patient is allowed a given number of "lifetime" visits. Finally, some insurers may require prior authorization after the initial visit or after a given number of visits. One should be familiar with guidelines of frequently encountered insurance companies in his or her setting.

- **Requiring a utilization review process:** Utilization review is a process where an insurance company employee, such as a nurse or case manager, reviews a patient's case and course of treatment to determine whether the care provided was medically necessary.[1]
- **Requiring case management:** Case managers direct patients to the most appropriate amount, duration, and type of health services and monitor medical outcomes. Insurance companies may employ case managers or may contract with an independent case management agency.
- **Using deductibles and copayments:** Many insurance policies include deductibles and copayments. These are payments provided to the health care providers that are the patient's responsibility and are part of the insurance coverage plan purchased by the patient. A deductible can range between a few hundred and thousands of dollars per year. Once the deductible is paid, then the remaining (or a portion of) money owed is covered by the insurance company. A copayment is a dollar amount paid by the patient each time a service is provided. For example, for therapy visits, a patient might be required to pay a $25 copayment per visit. Copayments and deductibles are very common among third-party payers, shifting more financial responsibility to the patient.

Casualty Insurance

Casualty insurance is a type of insurance that protects an individual who or company that might be responsible for an injury to another person(s).[25] An example is worker's compensation, which is an insurance program that protects a business in the event of an employee sustaining an injury on the job. Claims filed on behalf of the worker are paid by the employer's worker's compensation insurance. These claims are usually handled by payers other than health insurance companies. Benefits under workers' compensation plans vary, depending on the insurance company.

Indemnity Insurance

Indemnity insurance reimburses the patient for his or her out-of-pocket medical expenses that are covered under the insurance policy.[25] In other words, the patient pays the provider out of pocket and submits a claim to his or her insurance company. The insurance company then reimburses the patient.

Cash-Based Payment

In first-party payment, or cash-based services, the patient pays the bill in full on each day that services are provided. There are more physical therapy clinics today than ever before that incorporate cash-based services along with third-party reimbursement or that operate totally through cash-based services. Cash-based services decrease dependence on third-party payers; place additional responsibility on the patient, including his or her role in the care; and eliminate stipulations on the type, amount, frequency, or duration of services.[26] In addition, cash-based services provide daily cash flow into the clinic. The disadvantage of this type of payment is that patients may not be able to afford physical therapy services and, in these cases, educating them on the value of physical therapy is critical.[26]

Documentation and Reimbursement

In 1966, Medicare and Medicaid began requiring physicians and other health care providers to document medical procedures to be reimbursed.[27] In 1997, Baeten[28] indicated that documentation is the "key to securing reimbursement." Physical therapy documentation should include the physical therapist's initial documentation, which includes the examination, evaluation, plan of care, daily notes, progress notes, re-evaluations or reassessments (as necessary), and a final discharge summary. The primary documentation role of the physical therapist assistant is writing daily notes. Requirements for daily documentation are dependent on the setting. Medicare Part B daily documentation requirements include the following: the date of service, the identification of the specific treatment provided that is consistent with what was billed, the total timed code minutes and treatment time, and the signature and professional designation of the individual who provided or supervised the services and the individuals who contributed.[29,30] When appropriate, daily notes should also include the following: patient self-report, adverse reactions to the intervention, communication with other providers, changes in clinical status, equipment provided, and/or any other relevant information that is appropriate.[29]

Daily notes should help to provide support to the overall "story" of the patient and the episode of care including medical necessity of treatment. In doing so, one should also document the following as appropriate, a comparison between the patient's current functional status and his or her functional status at the initial evaluation; impairments and functional deficits in clear, concise, objective, and measurable language; the assistance provided, distinguishing between verbal and physical assistance; patient updates in a manner consistent with those on the initial evaluation; an explanation of why progress might be slower than expected; adequate information to support the medical necessity or rational for each treatment/procedure on every date it was billed; and evidence that the services required the unique skills of a therapist or supervision by a therapist.[31]

When documenting, one should always keep in mind that payment could depend upon information that is provided in the documentation. It is not enough to write, "patient is improving," "tolerated well," or "skilled services needed." Rather, be specific in describing subjective and objective changes, the skill(s) provided to the patient, how the interventions are bringing about change, and the reason for treatment.

REFERENCES

1. American Physical Therapy Association. *Glossary of payment terms.* APTA website. http://www.apta.org/Payment/Glossary/. Updated April 11, 2011. Accessed July 14, 2017.
2. *Definition of social insurance.* BusinessDictionary website. http://www.businessdictionary.com/definition/social-insurance.html. Accessed July 14, 2017.
3. Social Security Administration. *Legislative history.* SSA website. https://www.ssa.gov/history/law.html. Accessed October 16, 2017.
4. Barry P. *Do you qualify for Medicare?* AARP website. http://www.aarp.org/health/medicare-insurance/info-04-2011/medicare-eligibility.html. Updated March 2016. Accessed July 15, 2017.
5. US Department of Health & Human Services Press Office. *The new Centers for Medicare & Medicaid Services [press release].* US Department of Health & Human Services web site. http://archive.hhs.gov/news/ press/2001pres/20010614a.html. Published June 14, 2001. Accessed July 15, 2017.
6. Centers for Medicare & Medicaid Services. *About CMS.* CMS.gov website. https://www.cms.gov/About-CMS/About-CMS.html. Accessed July 15, 2017.
7. Kreis D. *What is the difference between Medicare Part A and Part B?* Medicare.com website. https://medicare.com/original-medicare/what-is-the-difference-between-medicare-part-a-part-b/. Updated November 17, 2015. Accessed July 15, 2017.
8. Centers for Medicare & Medicaid Services. *What is a MAC.* CMS.gov website. https://www.cms.gov/Medicare/Medicare-Contracting/ Medicare-Administrative-Contractors/What-is-a-MAC. html. Updated October 31, 2016. Accessed July 15, 2017.
9. Centers for Medicare & Medicaid Services. *Prospective Payment System—sgeneral information.* CMS.gov website. https://www.cms. gov/medicare/medicare-fee-for-service-payment/prospmedicarefeesvcpmtgen/index.html. Updated May 19, 2015. Accessed July 15, 2017.
10. Centers for Medicare & Medicaid Services. *Glossary.* CMS.gov website. https:// www.cms.gov/apps/glossary/default.asp. Updated May 14, 2006. Accessed July 15, 2017.
11. Centers for Medicare & Medicaid Services. *Skilled nursing facility PPS.* CMS.gov website. https://www.cms.gov/Medicare/MedicareFee-for-Service-Payment/SNFPPS/index.html?redirect=/ SNFPPS/01_overview.asp. Updated July 31, 2013. Accessed July 15, 2017.
12. Centers for Medicare & Medicaid Services. *Long-term care facilty resident assessment Instrument 3.0 user's manual [version 1.14].* CMS.gov website. https://downloads.cms.gov/files/MDS30-RAI-Manual-V114-October-2016.pdf. October 2016. Accessed July 15, 2017.
13. Centers for Medicare & Medicaid Services. *Inpatient rehabilitation facility PPS.* CMS.gov website. https://www.cms.gov/Medicare/ Medicare-Fee-for-Service-Payment/InpatientRehabFacPPS/ index.html?redirect=/InpatientRehabFacPPS/01_overview. asp%20updated%20 4/16/2013. Updated April 16, 2013. Accessed July 15, 2017.
14. *About the FIM System.* Uniform Data System for Medical Rehabilitation website. https://www.udsmr.org/WebModules/FIM/Fim_About.aspx. Accessed July 15, 2017.
15. Centers for Medicare & Medicaid Services. *OASIS overview.* CMS.gov website. https://www.cms.gov/Medicare/Quality-Initiatives-Patient-Assessment-Instruments/OASIS/Background.html. Updated March 5, 2012. Accessed October 16, 2017.
16. Centers for Medicare & Medicaid Services. *Home health PPS.* CMS.gov website. https://www.cms.gov/medicare/medicare-fee-for-service-payment/homehealthpps/index.html. Updated July 18, 2016. Accessed July 15, 2017.
17. Centers for Medicare & Medicaid Services. *Medicare Physician Fee Schedule overview.* CMS.gov website. https://www.cms.gov/ apps/physician-fee-schedule/. Updated July 3, 2017. Accessed July 15, 2017.
18. *RBRVS overview.* American Medical Association website. https://www.ama-assn.org/rbrvs-overview. Accessed July 15, 2017.
19. Smith TM. *Making sense of MACRA: a glossary of new Medicare terms.* AMA Wire website. https://wire.ama-assn.org/practice-management/making-sense-macra-glossarynew-medicare-terms. Published December 5, 2016. Accessed July 15, 2017.
20. American Physical Therapy Association. *FAQ: MACRA and Alternative Payment Models.* APTA website. http://www.apta.org/Payment/ Medicare/MACRA/FAQAPMs/. Updated November 2016. Accessed July 14, 2017.
21. *Medicare Bundled Payment for Care Improvement (BPCI) Initiative.* American Physical Therapy Association website. http://www.apta.org/BPCI/. Updated March 23, 2016. Accessed July 15, 2017.
22. Centers for Medicare & Medicaid Services. *Advance Beneficiary Notice of Noncoverage.* CMS.gov website. https://www.medicare. gov/claims-and-appeals/medicare-rights/abn/advancenotice-of-noncoverage.html. Accessed July 14, 2017.
23. *Program history.* Medicaid.gov website. https://www.medicaid.gov/about-us/program-history/index.html. Accessed July 15, 2017.
24. *Managed care.* MedlinePlus website. https://medlineplus.gov/managedcare.html. Updated December 31, 2016. Accessed July 15, 2017.
25. American Physical Therapy Association: *The Reimbursement Resource Guide.* Alexandria, VA: APTA; 2002.
26. Elliott C. *Responding to cost shifts.* PT in Motion. 2009;May. www.apta.org/PTinMotion/2009/5/GovernmentAffairs/.
27. Inaba M, Jones SL. Medical documentation for third-party payers. *Phys Ther.* 1977;57(7):791-794.
28. Baeten AM. *Documentation: the reviewer perspective.* Top Geriatr Rehabil. 1997;13(1):14-22.
29. *Medicare Part B documentation requirements.* APTA website. http://www.apta.org/Documentation/MedicarePartB/. Updated September 24, 11, 2017. Accessed July 15, 2017.
30. Centers for Medicare & Medicaid Services. *Medicare Benefit Policy Manual. Chapter 15 - covered medical and other expenses.* CMS.gov website. https://www.cms.gov/Regulations-and-Guidance/Guidance/Manuals/Downloads/bp102c15.pdf. Updated July 11, 2017. Accessed July 15, 2017.
31. United Government Services LLC. *Best documentation: concise and complete.* Presented at: Medicare Outpatient Therapy Services Educational Seminar; May 17, 2004; Flatwoods, WV.

Review Questions

1. In your own words, define reimbursement.

2. Who are the different parties responsible for the financial management of a patient's medical care? What is meant by third-party payment?

3. Describe the 4 types of insurance outlined in the chapter (social, managed care, casualty, and indemnity).

4. What are the major differences between Medicare Part A and Medicare Part B? What is Part C? What is Part D?

5. What is the difference between Medicare and Medicaid?

6. What strategies are used by managed care organizations to contain or lower costs? Give a brief description of each.

7. Define cash-based payment. What are some advantages and disadvantages of cash-based services?

8. List some ways that you can create documentation that has the potential to maximize reimbursement.

9. What are phrases to avoid using in documentation that will help in maximizing reimbursement?

10. Talk with a local clinician about the different types of insurance often accepted by his or her facility. What are the reimbursement guidelines? Try to identify examples of managed care plans and their guidelines.

Chapter 12

Legal and Ethical Considerations for Physical Therapy Documentation

Mia L. Erickson, PT, EdD, CHT, ATC

KEY TERMS Abuse | American Physical Therapy Association | American Society for Healthcare Risk Management | Centers for Medicare & Medicaid Services | Electronic protected health information | Fraud | Health Insurance Portability and Accountability Act of 1996 | Incident report | Informed consent | Privacy rule | Protected health information | Risk management | Secretary rule | US Department of Health & Human Services

KEY ABBREVIATIONS APTA | ASHRM | CMS | ePHI | HHS | HIPAA | PHI

Chapter Objectives

After reading this chapter, the reader will be able to do the following:

1. Describe federal legislation related to privacy and confidentiality.
2. Differentiate between the Health Insurance Portability and Accountability Act of 1996 (HIPAA) Privacy Rule and HIPAA Security Rule.
3. Compare ethical and legal responsibilities for maintaining confidentiality.
4. Define fraud and abuse.
5. Explain the purpose of risk management.
6. Realize the importance of informed consent.
7. Give reasons for filing an incident report.
8. Outline different agencies' responsibilities in establishing rules for documentation.

As previously indicated, documentation is an important part of being a health care provider. When individuals consider becoming a physical therapist or a physical therapist assistant, they usually do not realize the documentation requirements or the importance. After being in practice for several years and treating a variety of patients, it will become impossible to recall the details of each patient encounter; therefore, the information you record while the details are fresh in your head, will be your reference material if ever necessary. You should document so that, if you read the chart several years later, you will be able to recall the patient.

Although a full review of legal and ethical requirements and implications for medical record keeping is beyond the scope of this chapter, it provides an overview of important legal and ethical matters relevant to physical therapy documentation that influence day-to-day physical therapist assistant practice, including patient privacy and confidentiality, fraud and abuse, and risk management.

Patient Privacy and Confidentiality

Privacy Act of 1974 (5 U.S.C. § 552a)

The Privacy Act of 1974[1] set forth federal guidelines precluding health care agencies or providers from releasing or disclosing medical records or medical information

Erickson ML, McKnight R. *Documentation Basics for the Physical Therapist Assistant, Third Edition* (pp. 119-125)

to any person without first obtaining written consent, or a written request, from the patient. The Privacy Act required that providers and their employees to be trained on rules for handling an individual's records, and administrative efforts were aimed at minimizing threats to maintaining patient confidentiality. This legislation also allowed the patient the right to obtain a copy of his or her medical records (charges can be applied) and to discuss the records with his or her provider in the presence of another individual of the patient's choosing. Failure to comply with this Privacy Act would result in civil action against the provider.

In a clinical environment, it is important to maintain and respect the privacy and confidentiality of all information related to patients and clients. When working, one should take care not to leave charts or computers in open areas where they are accessible to people walking by, and one should be careful not to dictate in an open area to avoid being heard by others. Written records should also be kept in a secure, locked location so that they are not accessible to unauthorized individuals. Computer monitors should "time out" after a brief period of nonuse and should be accessible to employees only. Clinics and hospitals are also likely to have policies preventing employees from taking medical records or computers out of the building. Although the Privacy Act of 1974 still holds true today, additional legislation has been passed to further restrict the release of an individual's health information and medical records, including those transmitted via electronic media.

Health Insurance Portability and Accountability Act of 1996

The electronic transmission of information, including billing and claims filing, was meant to simplify some administrative processes; however, it also increased the risks of violating patient privacy and breaching confidentiality. In response, Congress mandated HIPAA (PL 104-191).[2] This legislation required the US Department of Health & Human Services (HHS) to implement standards for performing electronic health care transactions, ensuring patient privacy provisions, and protecting personally identifiable health information.[3] To fulfill the HIPAA requirement, the HHS published the HIPAA Privacy Rule and the HIPAA Security Rule.[4] Modifications to HIPAA were released in 2013.[5]

HIPAA Privacy Rule

The HIPAA Privacy Rule, also known as the HIPAA *Standards for Privacy of Individually Identifiable Health Information*, establishes national standards to protect, use, and disclose certain health information, called protected health information (PHI).[6] PHI includes both personal health information and individually identifiable health information. PHI includes demographic data and information related to past, present, or future physical or mental health or condition; the health care provided to the individual; past, present, and future payment for the provision of health care to the individual; and any information that could be used to identify an individual.[6]

Covered entities, or those who are required to follow HIPAA regulations, include the following: (1) health plans such as insurance companies, Medicare, and Medicaid; (2) health care providers who transmit electronic information such as claims, benefit eligibility inquiries, referral authorization requests, or other transactions for which the HHS has established standards; and (3) health care clearinghouses, or entities that process information that they receive in a nonstandard format into a standard format.[3,7] Other entities covered under the HIPAA legislation include contractors or other personnel who are not employees of the covered entity but will have access to the data while providing services to the covered entity. These associates are called business associates and include: billing companies that help in processing claims, companies that administer health plans; outside lawyers, accountants, or information technology specialists; and companies that destroy medical records.[7] Electronic media refers to the Internet, intranets and extranets, leased lines, dial-up lines, private networks, or transmissions occurring through magnetic tape, disk, or compact disk.[8]

In addition to protecting identifiable health information, the Privacy Rule requires covered entities to create written privacy policies and procedures.[3] Covered entities must also make available to patients explanations of their privacy rights, allow easier patient access to medical records (although charges may be applied), provide employee privacy training, and appoint a privacy officer. Under the Privacy Rule, however, providers are allowed to supply information to insurance companies and third-party payers when seeking reimbursement, and they are permitted to discuss information with other health care providers who are caring for the patient without any additional written consent from the patient. Information provided to these entities should be on a minimum necessary basis, meaning that providers should only disclose the minimum necessary information relevant to accomplish the purpose.[3,8]

HIPAA Security Rule

The HIPAA Security Rule, or the Security Standards for the Protection of Electronic Protected Health Information, was finalized after the Privacy Rule. It applies to the same covered entities as the Privacy Rule. The Health Information Technology for Economic and Clinical Health (HITECH) Act of 2009 expanded the responsibilities of the business associates under the Privacy and Security Rules.[4] The Security Rule protects a subset of information covered by the Privacy Rule that includes all identifiable health information that a covered entity creates, receives, maintains, or transmits in electronic form, or electronic protected health information (ePHI). In addition, it provides necessary administrative, physical, and technical safeguards that must be put into place to protect ePHI.[4] Under the Security Rule, covered entities must designate a security officer, implement audit and integrity policies, train and supervise employees on the Security Rule, physically safeguard workspaces such as limiting access to facilities and workstations, and implement policies and procedures for altering and destroying ePHI.[4] HIPAA does not replace any state laws, nor does it preclude states from having more restrictive legislation for protecting patient privacy. HIPAA merely provides minimum acceptable standards for maintaining and protecting patient privacy.[8]

Both physical therapists and physical therapist assistants have legal and ethical responsibilities for maintaining confidentiality and patient privacy. Legal responsibilities are outlined in the HIPAA legislation and can be further defined by state laws. Failure to comply with the law can result in civil and/or criminal action. Ethical responsibilities are generally determined by professional associations through the development and implementation of a code of ethics. The ethical responsibilities of a physical therapist assistant have been identified in the American Physical Therapy Association (APTA) *Standards of Ethical Conduct for the Physical Therapist Assistant*[9] and interpreted in the *APTA Guide for Conduct of the Physical Therapist Assistant.*[10] Standard 2, Part D, indicates that physical therapist assistants shall protect confidential patient information and provide it only when appropriate and allowed by law (in collaboration with the physical therapist).[9]

Fraud and Abuse

Health care fraud can cost taxpayers billions of dollars.[11] Insurance fraud can be defined as intentionally billing an insurance company, Medicare, or other third-party payer for services that were not provided or billing for an item or service that has higher reimbursement than the service provided. Insurance fraud is both illegal and unethical. It is a crime, and it exposes individuals or entities to potential criminal and civil liability and may lead to imprisonment, fines, and penalties.[11] Medicare beneficiaries are encouraged to report suspected accounts of fraudulent activity to the Office of Inspector General. The *Standards of Ethical Conduct for the Physical Therapist Assistant*[9] and the *APTA Guide for Conduct of the Physical Therapist Assistant*[10] put forth that physical therapist assistants should demonstrate integrity, including providing truthful and accurate information and discouraging misconduct. Keeping with this responsibility, it is also the physical therapist assistant's duty to report any unethical or illegal acts, including knowledge of fraudulent billing practices.[9,10]

Another improper billing procedure is abuse. *Abuse* includes practice that is not consistent with providing patients with services that are medically necessary, meeting professional standards, and being priced fairly.[11] Abuse is when a provider bills for items that are not necessary, charges excessively for a service or supply, or misuses billing codes.[11] Abuse is also illegal and punishable by law. Abuse differs from fraud in that abuse includes improper billing procedures such as upcoding, whereas fraud includes intentionally billing for services not provided.[11] The terms fraud and abuse are often used interchangeably; however, they are very different.

Risk Management

A growing concern in litigious times and societies is risk management. Risk management involves understanding, analyzing, and addressing risk to make sure that organizations achieve their objectives.[12] Health care facilities or entities that would provide health or health-related services to patients or clients have made significant strides in developing Enterprise Risk Management programs.[13] The American Society for Healthcare Risk Management (ASHRM) has adopted the following definition: "Enterprise risk management in healthcare promotes a comprehensive framework for making risk management decisions which maximize value protection and creation by managing risk and uncertainty and their connections to total value."[13] According to the ASHRM, risk management involves much more than patient safety and includes a variety of areas such as documentation, credentialing, staffing, marketing, sales, media relations, fraud and abuse, recruitment, retention, the electronic health record, and facilities management, to name a few. Risk falls into 8 domains, or categories, including operational, clinical/patient safety, strategic, financial, human capital, legal/regulatory, technology, and hazard. Documentation falls into the operational domain.[13]

Facilities are likely to have risk managers, or risk management departments, whose responsibilities include minimizing potential risks for those who are involved with patient/client management and for those who might come into contact with the facility, as a patient, visitor, or employee. Risk managers identify factors that create risks that are internal or external to the organization and either create or minimize risks.[13] For example, risk managers investigate complaints or concerns as they are brought forth, usually by patients. An important aspect of their investigation is examining the patient record and available documentation to assure that the standard of care was met.

Informed Consent

Two important risk management documents that physical therapist assistants should be aware of are informed consent documents and incident reports. Informed consent is a process by which a treating health care provider discloses appropriate information to a competent patient so that the patient makes a voluntary choice, agreeing to or rejecting a specified treatment.[14] When patients lack competence to make decisions about their health care, a substitute decision maker is sought.[14] Many people think of informed consent as a form that is signed at the onset of treatment, and, while it is true that patients and clients sign forms that indicate consent to treatment, informed consent is a process that allows the provider to give details regarding the treatment, including the risks and benefits, and allows the patient to ask questions prior to making a decision as to reject or accept the proposed treatment.[15] The process of informed consent can be considered a patient safety issue and is considered a fundamental principle of health care.[15]

The goal of informed consent is to allow the patient the opportunity to be an informed participant in his or her health care decisions.[16] The process involves communicating the following elements: (1) the nature of the decision or procedure; (2) reasonable alternatives; (3) relevant risks, benefits, and uncertainties related to each procedure or alternative; (4) assessment of understanding; (5) acceptance of the intervention by the patient.[16] The process should be applied to all health care interventions.[15]

The physical therapist is legally and ethically responsible for obtaining informed consent prior to providing any intervention. However, the physical therapist assistant might need to obtain informed consent if he or she is initiating a new modality or exercise, as instructed by the physical therapist. It is necessary to stay abreast of literature describing the indications and contraindications of various interventions that you will be providing. In addition, you should be able to describe to patients the risks, benefits, and alternatives to interventions you perform.

Incident Report

An incident report is a report filed whenever an unexpected event occurs.[17] It involves the identification of the incident and the preparation of a report by personnel who are directly involved in the process in question at the time of the discovery of the event.[18] Events occur in the following 3 categories: (1) adverse outcomes to a treatment that has been provided (eg, burn, fall), (2) procedural breakdowns (eg, confidentiality breaches), and (3) catastrophic events (eg, performing a procedure on the wrong body part).[18] Incident reports are filed with the risk management department and are not recorded in the patient's medical chart.

Documentation Requirements

The Centers for Medicare & Medicaid Services (CMS) has set forth policies requiring health care facilities (inpatient, outpatient, and home health) seeking reimbursement from Medicare and Medicaid to maintain documentation to support the services provided and billed. The most current documentation guidelines for Medicare can be found on the CMS website in the *Medicare Benefit Policy Manual.*[19] They are available for inpatient rehabilitation facilities (Chapter 1), home health services (Chapter 7), skilled nursing facilities (Chapter 8), and outpatient facilities (Chapter 15); however, these are CMS's requirements and can only be applied to Medicare beneficiaries. Nevertheless, private insurance companies or other reimbursing agencies often follow Medicare and may have similar requirements.

State Practice Acts

Both physical therapists and physical therapist assistants are bound by practice acts in the state(s) where they provide care to patients. Each state has different regulations for physical therapist and physical therapist assistant practice, some more restrictive than others. The state practice acts may outline requirements for physical therapist and physical therapist assistant documentation. The Federation of State Boards of Physical Therapy has provided a website with links to state licensing agencies and state practice acts. This can be found at http://www.fsbpt.org/FreeResources/LicensingAuthoritiesContactInformation.aspx. One should become familiar with the practice act for any state where elements of patient/client management are provided.

American Physical Therapy Association

The APTA has published recommendations for appropriate documentation that can be used as resources. These include *Guidelines: Physical Therapy Documentation of Patient/Client Management*[20] and "Defensible Documentation for Patient/Client Management."[21] Although the national association represents physical therapy practitioners across the country, it is important to point out that physical therapists and physical therapist assistants must first be in compliance with their state practice acts. In addition, documentation requirements and guidelines are dynamic and tend to change as the health care system evolves. One has a professional responsibility to stay attuned to important changes in documentation requirements and, from a legal perspective, to comply with the state's practice act.

References

1. *Privacy Act of 1974.* US Department of Justice website. https://www.justice.gov/opcl/privacy-act-1974. Updated July 17, 2015. Accessed July 15, 2017.
2. The Health Insurance Portability and Accountability Act of 1996. *Public Law 104-191.* 104th Congress. https://www.gpo.gov/fdsys/pkg/PLAW-104publ191/html/PLAW-104publ191.htm. Accessed July 15, 2017.
3. US Department of Health & Human Services. Office of Civil Rights Policy Brief. *Summary of the HIPAA Privacy Rule.* US Department of Health & Human Services website. http://www.hhs.gov/sites/default/files/privacysummary.pdf. Updated May 2003. Accessed July 15, 2017.
4. US Department of Health & Human Services. *Summary of the HIPAA Security Rule.* US Department of Health & Human Services website. https://www.hhs.gov/ hipaa/for-professionals/security/laws-regulations/index. html?language=es. Reviewed July 26, 2013. Accessed July 15, 2017.

5. Crandall D. *Key provisions of the HIPAA Final Rule.* APTA website. http:// www.apta.org/PTinMotion/2013/5/ComplianceMatters/. Updated 2013. Accessed November 21, 2016.
6. US Department of Health & Human Services. *Summary of the HIPAA Privacy Rule.* US Department of Health & Human Services website http://www.hhs.gov/hipaa/for-professionals/privacy/laws-regulations/index.html. Reviewed July 26, 2013. Accessed July 15, 2017.
7. US Department of Health & Human Services. *Your rights under HIPAA.* US Department of Health & Human Services website https://www.hhs.gov/hipaa/for-individuals/ guidance-materials-for-consumers/index.html. Reviewed February 1, 2017. Accessed July 15, 2017.
8. Ravitz KS. The HIPAA privacy final modified rule. *PT Magazine.* 2002; November.
9. American Physical Therapy Association. *Standards of Ethical Conduct for the Physical Therapist Assistant.* HOD S0609-20-18. http://www.apta.org/uploadedFiles/APTAorg/About_Us/Policies/Ethics/StandardsEthicalConductPTA.pdf. Accessed July 15, 2017.
10. American Physical Therapy Association Ethics and Judicial Committee. *APTA Guide for Conduct of the Physical Therapist Assistant.* APTA website. http://www.apta.org/uploadedFiles/ APTAorg/Practice_and_Patient_Care/Ethics/ GuideforConductofthePTA.pdf. Updated September 4, 2013. Accessed July 15, 2017.
11. Centers for Medicare & Medicaid Services. *Medicare fraud & abuse: prevention, detection, and reporting.* CMS.gov website. https://www. cms.gov/Outreach-and-Education/Medicare-LearningNetwork-MLN/MLNProducts/downloads/Fraud_and_Abuse.pdf. Published October 2016. Accessed July 15, 2017.
12. *About risk management.* Institute of Risk Management website. https://www.theirm.org/about/risk-management/. Accessed July 15, 2017.
13. Carroll RL, Hoppes M, Hagg-Rickert S, et al. *Enterprise risk management: a framework for success.* American Society for Healthcare Risk Management website. http://www.ashrm.org/resources/patient-safety-portal/pdfs/ERM-WhitePaper-8-29-14-FINAL.pdf. Accessed July 15, 2017.
14. Appelbaum PS. Assessment of patients' competence to consent to treatment. *N Engl J* Med. 2007;357:1834-1840.
15. Cordasco KM. Chapter 39. *Obtaining informed consent from patients: brief update review.* In: Shekelle PG, Wachter RM, Pronovost PJ, et al. *Making Healthcare Safer II: An Updated Critical Analysis of the Evidence for Patient Safety Practices. AHQR Publication No. 13-E001-EF.* Rockville, MD: Agency for Healthcare Quality and Research (US); March 2013. https://archive.ahrq.gov/research/findings/evidence-based-reports/ptsafetyII-full.pdf. Accessed July 15, 2017.
16. De Bord J. Informed consent. *Ethics in Medicine.* University of Washington School of Medicine website. http://depts.washington.edu/bioethx/topics/consent.html#endref. Updated March 7, 2014. Accessed July 15, 2017.
17. Nurses Service Organization. *Why incident reports are a must.* Nurses Service Organization website. http://www.nso.com/risk-education/individuals/articles/Why-Incident-Reports-Are-A-Must. Updated 2016. Accessed November 29, 2016.
18. Wald H, Shojania KG. Chapter 4. *Incident reporting.* Agency for Healthcare Research and Quality website. https://archive.ahrq.gov/research/findings/evidence-based-reports/services/quality/er43/ptsafety/chapter4.html. Reviewed 2001. Accessed July 15, 2017.
19. Centers for Medicare & Medicaid Services. *Medicare Benefit Policy Manual.* Publication Number 100-02. https://www.cms.gov/Regulations-and-Guidance/Guidance/Manuals/Internet-Only-Manuals-IOMs-Items/CMS012673.html?DLPage=1&DLEntries=10&DLSort=0&DLSortDir=ascending. Accessed July 15, 2017.
20. American Physical Therapy Association. *Guidelines: Physical Therapy Documentation of Patient/Client Management.* BOD G03-05-16-41. https://www.apta.org/uploadedFiles/APTAorg/About_Us/Policies/BOD/Practice/DocumentationPatientClientMgmt.pdf. Updated December 14, 2009. Accessed July 15, 2017.
21. American Physical Therapy Association. *Defensible Documentation for Patient/Client Management.* APTA website. http:// www.apta.org/Documentation/DefensibleDocumentation/. Updated December 8, 2015. Accessed July 15, 2017.

Review Questions

1. What guidelines did the Privacy Act of 1974 establish?

2. What was the rationale for developing the HIPAA Privacy and Security Rules?

3. What are the requirements for health care providers under the HIPAA Privacy and Security Rules?

4. How do HIPAA's Privacy and Security Rules affect state law?

5. What is your ethical responsibility regarding confidentiality and documentation? Is this different from your legal responsibility? Why or why not?

6. Differentiate between fraud and abuse. Give an example of each.

7. What are your ethical responsibilities related to fraud and abuse?

8. Define risk management.

9. What is the role of risk managers?

10. How is documentation important to risk managers?

11. When seeking informed consent from a patient, what are the key pieces of information that should be provided to the patient?

12. Give 3 examples (other than those listed in the text) of when a physical therapist assistant would need to file an incident report.

13. What state and federal government agencies are responsible for setting guidelines for medical record documentation?

14. To what document(s) can you refer to find information regarding physical therapy documentation in your state?

15. Investigate the physical therapy practice act for documentation requirements in your state. How does it compare with the Federation of State Boards of Physical Therapy's model practice act?

Chapter 13

Documentation Across the Curriculum

Mia L. Erickson, PT, EdD, CHT, ATC and Tracy Rice, PT, MPH, NCS

Chapter Objectives

After reading this chapter, the reader will be able to do the following:

1. Create documentation based on information provided in the scenario.
2. Integrate documentation into physical therapy content areas.
3. Document objective data from tests and measures and patient functional performance.
4. Identify parts of a physical therapist evaluation that are important for noting in physical therapist assistant documentation.
5. Compare patient subjective and objective data and functional performance between an initial note and interim note.
6. Create documentation that shows a change in patient status between the initial documentation and the interim documentation.
7. Create an appropriate assessment and plan after reading the subjective and objective data.

The goal of this chapter is to provide the reader with more examples and to practice creating documentation. The chapter is organized by topics frequently covered in a physical therapist assistant curriculum. This includes a variety of physical therapy content areas and settings. Each topic or section provides additional documentation examples. There are examples that only require the rewriting of a few pieces of information to make them suitable for entry into a medical record, likewise, there are other examples that include an entire treatment session and require the rewriting of all of the information for an entire chart entry. Finally, there are examples that require the creation of the assessment and/or plan sections of the SOAP (subjective, objective, assessment, and plan) note based on the available information or after referring to the patient's initial note that has been provided. For all examples, write clearly and concisely, using appropriate abbreviations, symbols (see Appendix), and medical terminology.

The following physical therapy content areas are included in this chapter:

- Goniometry
- Strength assessment
- Therapeutic exercises
- Transfers
- Tilt table
- Wheelchair management
- Gait training
- Wound care
- Chronic obstructive pulmonary disease/vital signs
- Traumatic brain injury
- Spinal cord injury (SCI)
- Cerebrovascular accident (CVA)
- Lower-extremity (LE) amputation/prosthetic devices

Erickson ML, McKnight R. *Documentation Basics for the Physical Therapist Assistant, Third Edition* (pp. 127-153)

- Musculoskeletal trauma
- Pediatric/orthotic devices
- General documentation practices

Goniometry

For each of the following, rewrite the information so that it would be appropriate for recording into a note. Include subjective, objective, assessment and plan where appropriate.

1. You are working on increasing range of motion (ROM) in a patient who had a bimalleolar fracture on the right ankle. After taking the following measurements, you decide that her active range of motion (AROM) goal has been met and that she should be reevaluated by the physical therapist. AROM on the right ankle was 10° dorsiflexion and 50° plantarflexion. The left has 15° dorsiflexion and 55° plantarflexion.
2. You take the following measurements from a patient who is 3 weeks' status post-right CVA with left hemiplegia. AROM on the right upper and lower extremities is within normal limits; however, you take the following AROM measurements on the left: shoulder: 45° flexion and abduction, 40° internal rotation, 60° external rotation; elbow: flexion 100° and extension 0°; wrist extension 0° and flexion 50°. For the left LE, you record the following: hip: flexion 120°, abduction 20°; knee flexion 130° and extension 0°; ankle dorsiflexion 0° and plantarflexion 50°.
3. The following measurements were taken from a patient on June 21, 2017: AROM: right wrist flexion 50°, extension 60°, supination 45°, pronation 45°, ulnar deviation 10°, and radial deviation 5°. On June 24, you record the following measurements for the same patient: AROM: right wrist flexion 62°, extension 65°, supination 55°, pronation 60°, ulnar deviation 15°, and radial deviation 10°. Organize the measurements for the note on June 24. Also, record your assessment for that day.
4. You are working with a patient who has multiple sclerosis. You record the following measurements: AROM measurements taken at the ankles: 0° dorsiflexion and 50° plantarflexion, at the knees: extension -20° and flexion 135°, at the hips: flexion 100°, and abduction 20°. Passive range of motion (PROM) measurements: ankles: 20° dorsiflexion, knees: 0° extension, and hips: 120° flexion. Use the following table to organize your information as you would enter it into an electronic medical record. Indicate "Not Tested" where there are no data.

AROM	**Right**	**Left**
Ankle dorsiflexion		
Ankle plantarflexion		
Knee extension		
Knee flexion		
Hip flexion		
Hip abduction		

PROM	**Right**	**Left**
Ankle dorsiflexion		
Ankle plantarflexion		
Knee extension		
Knee flexion		
Hip flexion		
Hip abduction		

Strength Assessment

Rewrite the following information so that it would be appropriate for recording into a medical record. **You will need to assign the appropriate muscle grade(s) based on the description provided.** Your supervising physical therapist has asked you to perform manual muscle testing on a patient. Your findings are as follows:

1. When assessing the patient's right upper extremity (UE), he is able to take moderate resistance in shoulder flexion, extension, and internal rotation. For shoulder abduction and external rotation, he is only able to take minimal resistance. Also, he is able to take moderate resistance with elbow flexion and extension. All muscle tests were performed in the antigravity position.
2. When assessing a patient's right LE, he is able to take minimal resistance with hip abduction; moderate resistance with hip flexion, hip extension, and hip lateral rotation; moderate resistance with knee flexion; normal resistance with hip adduction, knee extension, and ankle dorsiflexion; and strong resistance with ankle plantarflexion. All muscle tests were performed in the antigravity position.
3. When assessing a patient's left UE, you must use the gravity-eliminated position for all testing. For shoulder adduction and medial rotation, the patient is able to complete full ROM in the gravity-eliminated position (he is only able to complete 25% of the range in the antigravity position), and he can hold the position on his own. When testing shoulder flexion, shoulder extension, shoulder abduction, and elbow extension, you record that he is only able to move through approximately 50% of the avail-

able ROM in the gravity-eliminated position. The patient is able to complete full available ROM and hold the gravity-eliminated position for elbow flexion, but he cannot hold against resistance. You are only able to palpate contractions for the shoulder lateral rotators and the wrist flexors and extensors in the gravity-eliminated positions.

4. When assessing the patient's left LE, he is able to complete full AROM and take minimal resistance in the antigravity position when testing hip extensors, hip adductors, and hip internal rotators. He is able to complete full AROM against gravity and is able to maintain the test position against moderate resistance for hip flexors and ankle plantarflexors. He is unable to complete full ROM against gravity with hip lateral rotators and knee extensors. You position him in the gravity-eliminated position, and he is able to complete only 50% of the available AROM for these motions. Only a palpable contraction can be noted with knee flexors and ankle dorsiflexors.

Therapeutic Exercises

Organize the following 3 cases into SOAP format and then answer the questions that follow.

Case 1. *You are working in the acute care hospital setting with an elderly woman who has suffered a right CVA. The supervising PT has asked you to assist with part of this patient's treatment today. The patient is cooperative and has no complaints. The patient indicates an improvement in motion in the involved extremities and an improvement in toileting. You perform passive and active assisted ROM to the patient's left extremities. The patient is not showing any signs of abnormal tone or signs of developing contractures. You perform 3 sets of 10 repetitions. You also provide manual resistance to the patient's right LE in proprioceptive neuromuscular facilitation D1 and D2 patterns. The patient performs 2 sets of 10 repetitions for the resisted ROM. Finally, you provide stretching to the patient's tight ankle plantarflexors bilaterally. You provide the stretch 5 times for each side, holding each stretch for 30 seconds. You will continue the same treatment the following day and progress as instructed by the PT. The treatment session lasted 12'.*

Case 2. *You just finished working with a patient receiving home health care who had a total knee arthroplasty 10 days ago. She was in her bed and performed exercises to work on ROM. She said that she had some pain (3/10) during the previous night, and she continues to have swelling that she feels is preventing her from bending her knee more. Her biggest complaints right now are not being able to sit normally, not being able to go up and down stairs, and not being able to drive due to the ROM limitations in the knee. Her AROM at the knee was 10° from full extension and 95° flexion. You had the patient perform 20 repetitions of heel slides, ankle dorsiflexion and plantar flexion, short arc knee extension exercises (0-45°), and active hip abduction and adduction. You also worked on gentle passive stretching to improve knee flexion while the patient was seated at the edge of the bed. She ambulated 50' twice with close supervision for balance and verbal cues for walker placement and sequencing, weight bearing as tolerated on the right with a standard walker. She stated that she felt good after the exercises, and her assistance level needed is decreasing. You tell her that you will see her in 2 days to continue the exercises and that you will progress them as she can tolerate. Active knee motion increased to 110° following the treatment and she could sit more comfortably. Total treatment time was 45'.*

Case 3. *You are working with a patient who had a rotator cuff repair 8 weeks ago. During the last session, you initiated resistive ROM exercises (isometric setting) to begin strengthening the deltoid. He returns to the clinic today and tells you that he has felt good since his last treatment and that he thinks that the isometric exercises are getting too easy. He thinks that he is able to dress and perform self-care with greater ease. He also notes improved ability to reach into overhead cabinets. After consulting the plan of care, you decide to progress the patient to using an exercise band (2 sets of 10 repetitions). While in the clinic that day, he begins shoulder flexion and internal and external rotation using the yellow exercise band. He also performs his usual routine including 20 repetitions of flexion and external rotation with a wand, scapular retraction and protraction, and active external and internal rotation in the side lying position. You also perform 20 repetitions of PROM for flexion, internal and external rotation, and abduction. After the treatment, he says that he feels good and that he thinks that the new exercises are not that hard. He will return next week, and his exercises will be progressed per the rotator cuff protocol and as he is able to tolerate. Total treatment time was 45'.*

1. From the 3 cases above, what pieces of information help you in determining the patient's response to the intervention?
2. Where should the patient's response to treatment be documented in the note?
3. In your notes, did you remember to include the skill that was provided to the patient? How?
4. In your notes, did you show the relationship between impairment and activity limitations and participation restrictions? Did you describe how the treatment was impacting the patient's activity limitations and participation restrictions?

Transfers

For each of the following, rewrite the information so that it would be appropriate for recording into a medical record.

1. The patient moved from the bed to the chair with 25% assistance provided by 1 PT. The stand pivot transfer was used.
2. The patient moved from the wheelchair to the floor using both of his upper extremities with supervision and verbal cueing from the PT.
3. The PT transferred the patient in the Hoyer lift from the bed to the wheelchair.
4. The patient moved supine to sit and sit to supine on the mat table with 50% of the assistance provided by the PT.
5. The patient required 50% of the PT's assistance when moving from the wheelchair to the mat table when transferring to the left (squat pivot transfer); however, she could transfer to the right with only 25% of assistance provided by the PT.
6. Your client is a 58-year-old woman who suffered a compound fracture of the right ankle 2 days ago. You are to teach her how to transfer effectively from the wheelchair to the bedside commode. She is non-weightbearing on the affected side and is wearing a plaster cast, immobilizing the foot and ankle. The patient is obese and requires moderate assistance of 2 people for transferring in and out of a bed to a wheelchair. She says that she is in severe pain (8/10) and is hesitant to participate. While using a walker, she is able to stand and doff her pants with minimal assistance, but still requires moderate assistance of 2 people to complete the transfer from the bed to the bedside commode due to fear of falling and difficulty maintaining non-weightbearing status.
7. You are working with a 68-year-old woman who is recovering from a brainstem CVA. Slide board transfer training with this patient has not gone well. She has made poor progress over the last 2 weeks, and the focus of treatment has changed to educating her husband on how to care for his wife. The supervising PT has asked you to begin Hoyer transfer training with the patient and her husband. The patient is disappointed that she has not made any significant improvements, but she continues to be motivated and upbeat with therapy. She has stated that she is "not going to give up." The husband required moderate assistance placing the Hoyer sling and setting up for the transfer, and needed minimal assistance during the transfer. The patient will be discharged to home with her husband as soon as he is able to care for her independently.
8. You are working with a 28-year-old male patient who is in rehab due to a T4 SCI with paraplegia. During this therapy session, you concentrate on working with the patient on his slide board transfers for 30'. The patient is able to perform wheelchair setup with minimal assistance of 1 to assist with weight shift and occasional verbal cues, but he requires moderate assistance with slide board placement. The patient requires maximal assistance with the transfer. The patient shares with you during therapy today that he is concerned about his family and how he is going to manage caring for his farm. The patient appears depressed and anxious during this session. While looking at the initial evaluation note, you notice that there is a goal for the patient to be independent in slide board transfers.
9. You are working with an inpatient with Guillain-Barré syndrome. He reports that he is doing better today. Exercises (3 sets of 10 reps) consisted of ankle pumps, active hip abduction, heel slides, bridging, and knee extension at the edge of the bed. After exercises, you work on transfers to the wheelchair, which is positioned next to the bed using a stand pivot transfer. The patient requires approximately 25% to 30% assistance from you, but you are able to provide this yourself without difficulty, although you do have to block his knees so they do not buckle due to weakness. After this, the patient transfers back to bed, but because of fatigue and bed height, he requires 50% to 60% assistance. He performs sit to and from supine with 50% assistance because of weakness. He is unable to lift his legs onto the bed from the floor. He is able to position himself in bed without the use of side rails while scooting and bridging with verbal cues. There is no improvement in the patient's ability to transfer from the previous day's note. You tell him that you will see him in the afternoon for gait in the therapy department.

Tilt Table

For each of the following, rewrite the information so that it would be appropriate for recording into a medical record. Include as many parts of the SOAP note as possible.

1. You are helping a 78-year-old patient who requires maximum assistance from 3 to 4 people to stand, and, upon standing, he complains of dizziness. The PT decides to begin standing activities on the tilt table. The patient has been sitting up in a wheelchair without any complaints or problems. The patient is able to tolerate getting to a full upright position and stay for 10 minutes before complaining of fatigue or dizziness. The patient's blood pressure readings remained 120/74 mm Hg for the full 10 minutes.
2. You are working with a 28-year-old patient who has a closed head injury and exhibits severe hypertonia. The PT asks you to use the tilt table to help manage LE spasticity. The patient tolerates the procedure without a change in blood pressure (110/76 mm Hg). The patient remains in the upright position for 20 minutes.
3. A 67-year-old man is recovering from a lengthy illness associated with acute respiratory failure, and

he is having consistent problems with orthostatic hypotension. The patient has had 2 previous tilt table treatments and was able to get up to approximately 45° before his blood pressure dropped significantly. At 0°, it was 108/68 mm Hg. At 45°, it was 92/58 mm Hg after 1 minute.

Wheelchair Management

For each of the following, rewrite the information so that it would be appropriate for recording into a medical record.

1. The patient worked on wheelchair propulsion on ramps and level surfaces for 30 minutes, including tile and carpet, and he is now able to propel independently on all surfaces and manage leg rests and brakes without cueing. Prior to today, he was requiring minimal assistance and verbal cues.
2. You are working with a 16-year-old patient with a T1 spinal cord lesion. The patient currently needs moderate assistance to perform transfers to and from the wheelchair with a slide board. The patient currently requires occasional verbal cues and minimal assistance to set up the slide board and prepare the wheelchair's arm and leg rests for safe mobility in and out.
3. The patient is a 24-year-old woman who was involved in a motor vehicle accident in which she sustained bilateral femur fractures. The patient has undergone surgery and is now being taught slide board transfers from the wheelchair to and from the bed. The patient requires moderate assistance for board setup and minimal assistance for managing the wheelchair parts. She needs moderate assistance from 2 people to transfer in and out of the wheelchair.
4. You are working with a 58-year-old patient with diabetes, a right above-knee amputation, and a left below-knee amputation. The patient has been assigned the following scores on the Functional Independence Measure (FIM).[1] Write the objective portion of your note so that levels of assistance correspond with the FIM scores. Bed, chair, and wheelchair transfers = 3; toilet, tub, and shower transfers = 2; wheelchair mobility = 4.
5. You are working with a patient who has a T3 complete spinal cord lesion with resultant paraplegia. He has been working on the slide board to transfer in and out of his wheelchair. Currently, he is requiring minimal assistance from the PT to set up and prepare the chair. He requires moderate assistance for the transfer. The ultimate goal is for him to be independent. You spend 20 minutes on transfer training. He has also been working on wheelchair mobility, including ramps, gravel, sidewalks, and carpet. He can perform all of these mobility skills with verbal cueing for weight shifting and occasional minimal assistance for trunk control. The goal for wheelchair mobility is also for independence (an additional 10 minutes is spent on wheelchair mobility). For the last part of the treatment session (20 minutes), you work on transferring from the wheelchair to the floor. He requires minimal assistance to go to the floor, but requires maximal assistance to get back into the chair. This goal is also for him to be independent. You notice on the initial evaluation note that the patient required maximal assistance of 2 people for all transfers and moderate assistance of 1 person for wheelchair mobility skills when he was admitted to the facility. The plan is to see him twice a day (in the morning for the above and in the afternoon for strengthening, stretching, and continued functional mobility).

Gait Training

For each of the following, rewrite the information so that it would be appropriate for recording into a SOAP note.

Parallel Bars

1. You assist a 76-year-old patient who underwent bilateral total knee arthroplasties to ambulate in the parallel bars. She is able to ambulate 10' with moderate assistance of 1 person requiring verbal cues for hand placement.
2. An 82-year-old patient with a right below-knee amputation is beginning gait training with his new prosthesis in the parallel bars. He is able to ambulate 20' with minimal assistance of 1 person. He required verbal cues to weight shift to the right.
3. A 45-year-old patient with multiple sclerosis has bilateral LE weakness, coordination problems, and balance deficits. The patient ambulates 20' in the parallel bars with moderate assistance from 1 person and verbal cueing for upright posture. He required manual assistance at the knees to prevent his knee from buckling bilaterally.

Crutches

1. You are working with a 46-year-old patient who underwent an arthroscopic surgery on his left LE to ambulate with crutches. He is allowed to weight bear as tolerated and needs minimal assistance from 1 person for ambulation on level surfaces (for 30 feet) and up and down 2 steps.
2. You are assisting a 26-year-old patient who suffered a right femur fracture to ambulate with crutches. The patient is non-weightbearing on the right LE. The patient has poor balance, but only requires minimal assistance from 1 person on level surfaces

and up and down steps. The patient can ambulate for 50 feet before requiring a rest break.

3. You are working alone with a 38-year-old woman with multiple sclerosis who recently underwent a right total knee arthroplasty. You are assisting the patient in ambulating with the Lofstrand crutches. The patient requires moderate assistance and is allowed to bear weight as tolerated. She can ambulate 25 feet before requiring a break due to fatigue. She has considerably decreased endurance and becomes short of breath easily. Respiratory rate increased from 15 to 25 respirations per minute after gait.

Cane

1. You are assisting a 64-year-old woman following a right CVA to ambulate with a hemi-cane. The patient requires moderate assistance from 1 person to ambulate 50'. She requires this assistance to advance her left leg and verbal cues to achieve heel strike with the left foot.
2. You are assisting a 78-year-old patient who suffered a left humerus fracture and is having mild balance deficits in learning to ambulate with a straight cane. The patient requires minimal assistance of 1 person due to balance deficits to ambulate 150' on level surfaces.
3. A 64-year-old patient who underwent a right total hip arthroplasty 6 weeks ago is ready to advance from using a walker to using a cane. After instructing the patient to use a cane, you provide contact guard assistance of 1 person and verbal cueing for proper sequencing to ambulate 75'.

Walker

1. You are assisting a 74-year-old patient who recently underwent a right total hip arthroplasty in learning to ambulate with a standard walker. The patient requires moderate assistance of 2 people and is allowed to weight bear as tolerated to walk 75 feet.
2. You are assisting an 84-year-old patient who fell and suffered a right wrist and right femur fracture. The patient underwent surgical fixation for the right femur and is partial weight bearing (50%) on the right LE. You assist her in ambulating with a standard walker with a UE platform. She requires moderate assistance for 25 feet and reminders that she can only place 50% of her weight on the involved LE.
3. You are assisting an 88-year-old patient who is recovering from pneumonia. She is deconditioned and has mild balance problems. Her endurance is poor, so she is only able to ambulate 25' before tiring and requiring a rest break. Following the activity, her oxygen saturation level was 91%. Prior to the activity, it was 98%. The patient only requires minimal assistance from 1 person and uses a wheeled walker. Her rate of perceived exertion as measured on the Borg Rating of Perceived Exertion Scale during the activity was 17/20.

Organize the following 3 cases into SOAP format and then answer the questions that follow:

Case 1. *You are assisting a 28-year-old man who underwent an open reduction and internal fixation surgery for a fractured femur now weight bearing as tolerated on the right. You are assisting this patient with crutch gait on level surfaces and steps for 30 minutes. The patient ambulates 300' on level surfaces and up and down 2 flights of steps independently and safely. The patient is ready for discharge. He voices that he wants to go home and is confident that he will be able to handle himself. You reference the initial evaluation documentation and see that the patient has met all of the goals established by the PT. He will be discharged to home in the next 1 to 2 days, and you think that home health would be a good idea for this patient.—*

Case 2. *You are working with a 67-year-old patient who underwent a left total hip replacement. The weightbearing status is weight bear as tolerated. You see the patient 2 days after the initial evaluation in the skilled nursing facility. Today, the patient walks with the walker 100 feet on a level surface and only requires contact guard assistance from 1 person. At the time of the initial evaluation, the patient needed minimal assistance. You also began stair training. The patient walked up and down 5 steps with the rail on the right side and a cane on the left and required constant verbal cues for sequencing and minimal assistance. The patient voices that he feels that he is ready to go home. The goals are for the patient to be independent with gait 200 feet and on stairs, since he will be home alone. You will continue to work on progressing the patient in gait and stairs so that he can return home.*

Case 3. *You have been working with a 72-year-old man who is recovering from a left CVA. The patient is working on gait in the parallel bars. The patient gets easily fatigued and is only able to take 5 to 6 steps at a time. The patient requires maximal assistance to ambulate and needs assistance advancing and placing his right leg and manual assistance at the knee. The patient voices that he is sure that he will never be able to walk again and says, "We are wasting our time."*

1. From the 3 cases above, what pieces of information help you in determining the patient's response to the intervention?
2. In the above note, how did you document the patient's response to treatment?
3. In your notes, did you describe the need for skilled services? How?
4. In your notes, is your clinical decision making apparent? Why or why not?
5. In your notes, did you describe how the impairments are impacting the patient's function? How?

Wound Care

For each of the following, rewrite the information so that it would be appropriate for recording into a medical record.

1. Upon removing the dressing, you notice minimal drainage on the dressing. The drainage present is yellow exudate.
2. The wound bed is necrotic and is entirely filled with black eschar.
3. The area around the wound is red. It feels warm. It is shiny, and there is also no hair around the wound.
4. After removing the previous day's dressing, you notice a "sweet" odor and a moderate amount of greenish drainage on the dressing.
5. Wound is 4 cm in length and 2 cm in width. The depth is 3 mm. There is tunneling 2 inches at 12:00, toward the head.
6. The wound is located at the distal aspect of the right lateral leg, just below the lateral malleolus. It has a moderate amount of reddish-brown drainage. It is 2 cm by 2 cm with no significant depth.
7. The wound is located on the top of the right foot. Edema is present in the foot and ankle. Figure 8 girth at the ankle is 20 cm on the right and 16 cm on the left. The periwound area is painful, red, and warm to the touch. The dorsal pedal pulse is present and is 1+ on the right and 2+ on the left.
8. The wound is on the anterior aspect of the left tibia. It is 3 cm in length and 4 cm in width. The depth is 5 mm. The wound is full thickness and irregularly shaped. It has 50% granulation and approximately 25% yellow slough. Part of the tibia and anterior tibialis are exposed. There is no odor present. Sensation is decreased to light touch on the left from the knee down. The treatment consisted of a warm water soak for 10' and dressing change using a hydrocolloid dressing to cover the wound.

Organize the following case into SOAP format:

You have been assigned a patient with a stage 3 open wound at the head of the right first metatarsal. The patient also has atherosclerosis, and diabetes mellitus. The patient complains of severe pain (7/10) and difficulty walking. Upon dressing removal, there is a minimal amount of nonmalodorous reddish-brown drainage from the wound bed. The wound bed is moist, and approximately 50% of the wound bed includes granulation tissue and 50% is covered with yellow adhered slough. The skin around the wound is red, warm to the touch, shiny, and swollen. The wound is an 4 cm × 2.4 cm oval-shaped wound. It is 1.5-cm deep. The patient has diminished sensation to light touch around the wound when compared bilateral. She is unable to feel the 10 g monofilament on the plantar surface of the right foot. Girth at the right metatarsophalangeal joints is 22 cm and 18 cm on the left. The right dorsal pedis pulse is present but diminished compared with the left, which is 2+. Treatment consisted of whirlpool at 98°F × 15 minutes to the right LE followed by debridement of a minimal amount of yellow slough from the wound bed. After the treatment, the wound was covered with saline-soaked gauze and wrapped with Kling. It appears to you that the amount of yellow slough in the wound bed is decreasing. The initial evaluation note states that there was approximately 75% yellow adhered slough when the patient began the episode of care, although there is not much change in wound size. The plan is to continue with wet to wet dressing treatment and to try to have the patient begin ambulating as the wound allows. You are going to talk to the PT about the possibility of acquiring specialized footwear for the patient to allow weight bearing without disrupting wound healing.

Chronic Obstructive Pulmonary Disease/Vital Signs

Organize the following information into a format for entry into a medical record. Determine what to include in the assessment and plan portions of the note. Try to incorporate evidence of the need for skilled care, a description of how the impairments are influencing function, the patient's response to interventions, and clinical problem solving.

You have been assigned a 74-year-old female patient who is deconditioned with a diagnosis of chronic obstructive pulmonary disease. The treatment plan from the initial evaluation note (performed yesterday) states that the patient will be seen twice daily for endurance exercises and gait training. Upon entering the room, the patient is holding an oxygen mask to her face and taking deep inspirations and short expirations. She complains of difficulty breathing and moving around because she "can't get her breath." She is on 8 L of oxygen at rest. A vital signs check before activity reveals the following: pulse 98 beats per minute, blood pressure 120/84 mm Hg, respirations 20 per minute, and oxygen saturation 92%. She agrees to participate in bedside exercise, and you spend 15 minutes working on her UE and LE AROM, assuring that her oxygen saturation level stays above 90%. After a rest break, she ambulates 30 feet from her bed to and from the bathroom with contact guard assistance for safety. She requires the oxygen mask with oxygen levels set at 8 L during gait. She requires supervision during toileting secondary to complaints of dizziness. She returns to her bed and transfers sit to supine with moderate assistance from 1 person. After exercises and gait, her vitals are as follows: pulse 108 beats per minute, blood pressure 124/84 mm Hg, respirations 24 per minute, and oxygen saturation 90%. During the initial examination, the patient was unable to ambulate because of her shortness of breath, and her resting vitals were as follows: pulse 104 beats per minute, blood pressure 120/88 mm Hg, respirations 24 per minute, and oxygen saturation 90% at rest.

Traumatic Brain Injury

Provided by Tracy Rice, PT, MPH, NCS

Organize the following information into an appropriate documentation format. Determine what to include in the assessment and plan. Try to incorporate evidence of the need for skilled care and link impairment to function, response to interventions, and clinical problem solving. After writing the note, consider what additional information could you include that would improve your note.

Your patient is a 17-year-old male in an inpatient rehabilitation facility. His diagnosis is diffuse axonal injury secondary to being ejected in a motor vehicle accident. He presents with left-side weakness, increased tone, and spasticity. The patient presents with extensor tone/pattern on the left LE and flexor tone/synergy on the left UE. He is alert, awake, and inconsistently cooperative. He is oriented to person only. He is unaware of his situation, time, and place. He inconsistently follows simple commands, is sometimes combative, and demonstrates a short attention span. He responds well to an established routine and automatic tasks. His treatment session consisted of the following activities. You worked on bed mobility in the patient's room. He performed rolling to the right with moderate assistance x 1 and rolling to the left with minimal assistance x 1 and the use of the bed rail. The patient performed supine to sit at the edge of the bed with moderate assistance x 1 and minimal assistance x 1 to maintain static sitting balance on the compliant bed surface. All bed mobility activities required verbal cues for sequencing. The patient performed a stand pivot transfer to the right from the bed to the wheelchair with moderate assistance x 1 and blocking of the left knee to prevent buckling. The patient propelled himself utilizing the right hemi-body to the therapy gym with verbal cues for sequencing the use of the wheelchair with the right UE and LE and for attention to task. In the gym, you worked on additional functional activities. The patient performed wheelchair to mat transfer to the left with maximal assistance via stand pivot with blocking of the left knee to promote extension and prevent buckling. The patient performed repetitive sit to stand from the mat table with moderate assistance x 1 with manual assistance at the left LE for extension during the sit to stand transition. The patient ambulated 50' with rollator platform front-wheeled walker with minimal assistance of 1 to support the left UE and to guide the rollator and maximal assistance of another for manual assistance for step initiation on the left, blocking of left knee during stance phase of gait and for postural control. The patient required verbal cues throughout the gait process for upright posture, both head and trunk control, attention to task, and to increase step on the right LE to encourage stance on the left LE. The patient required his left ankle to be ace wrapped into dorsiflexion secondary to extensor tone and foot drop. He tolerated the standing frame for 45 minutes where you performed PROM to the left UE. You performed PROM to the shoulder in all planes of movement, the elbow, the wrist, and the hand, where you emphasized long finger extensors and increasing the web space and thumb abduction. Overall, you feel that the patient is progressing and meeting his goals, but you continue to feel that he would benefit from inpatient acute rehabilitation.

Spinal Cord Injury

Provided by Tracy Rice, PT, MPH, NCS

Organize the following information so that it would be appropriate for entry into a medical record. Determine what to include in the assessment and plan portions of the note. Try to incorporate evidence of the need for skilled care and link impairment to function, response to interventions, and clinical problem solving. After writing the note, consider what additional information could you include that would improve your note.

Your patient is a 21-year-old man with a T6 complete SCI as a result of a motor vehicle accident. The patient is alert and oriented to person, place, time, and situation. He has been in acute rehabilitation for the last 2 weeks. He is making good progress, and today his treatment consists of transfer training and functional activities in preparation for discharge to home. The patient performs repetitive wheelchair to mat and mat to wheelchair transfers. The patient performs them via multiple techniques to determine the most efficient and safest transfer technique and for functional endurance and strength training. The patient performs the transfer via lateral scoot with very close supervision to contact guard assistance for wheel clearance. He performs that transfer repetitively x 5. Throughout the transfer sequence, the patient required verbal cues for technique. Verbal cues for scooting further forward in the chair, emphasizing the head-hip relationship, greater push through the UEs for better clearance, leaning forward and foot placement. He also performed wheelchair to mat and mat to wheelchair utilizing the transfer board with supervision and verbal cues for technique for board placement, head-hip relationship, and scooting with clearance rather than sliding on the board to protect his skin integrity. This technique was repeated 5 times. The patient performed short sitting on the edge of mat with supervision. The patient worked on dynamic sitting balance activities to encourage moving center of gravity over base of support: ball tossing, batting a balloon, reaching to the floor to don and doff shoes. All balance activities were performed for 15 minutes as an endurance activity with close supervision to occasional contact guard assistance for loss of balance. The patient performed sit to supine with supervision with for sequencing technique for efficiency. Once the patient was in supine, he worked on rolling left and right with supervision and verbal cues for technique with UE momentum and LE positioning. He worked on supine to long sitting with contact guard assistance x 1 and verbal cues to maintain body weight anteriorly during the transition and then to prop himself up on extended arms. He performed dynamic balance activities in long sitting to promote unsupported sitting without the use of bilateral UEs to allow for independent dressing. The patient performed ball tossing, batting a balloon, and lower body dressing to promote moving center of gravity over base of support in long sitting. The patient transitioned to ring sitting and performed the same balance activities to promote independent sitting and independent self-care. The patient transitioned from ring sitting into prone lying with minimal assistance for LE management. From prone lying, the patient transitioned into side lying and then into sitting on the edge of the mat with minimal assistance and verbal cues for sequencing through the transitions. The therapy session ended by transferring from edge of mat to wheelchair via lateral scoot with contact guard assistance x 1. The patient demonstrated good motivation and cooperation throughout the session, despite having expressed some feelings of depression and longing to go home. His affect throughout is slightly flat, but he continues to be motivated and to perform all activities asked of him despite the difficulty. Based on the treatment session, you feel that the patient needs to continue to work on his transfer technique secondary to some technique flaws resulting in inefficiencies and not always clearing the surface in which he is transferring to, which places him at risk for skin breakdown.

Cerebrovascular Accident

The following is the initial examination/evaluation documentation for a patient recently admitted to an inpatient rehabilitation hospital. Use it to help you complete the following 2 entries for a medical record. Include the following in your notes:

- Write the assessment and plan portions of the notes based on available information provided in the initial evaluation documentation.
- Write your notes to maximize reimbursement.
- Be specific when documenting your interventions (include patient education, coordination or communication with other disciplines, and procedural intervention).

When you are finished, answer the following questions:

1. When writing the plan, what would be appropriate based on the initial plan of care provided and the patient's status?
2. Look at the patient's functional level for your notes. What would be corresponding FIM scores for this patient on these dates of service?

Cerebrovascular Accident Case

Pr: (L) CVA with (R) hemiplegia 1 week ago; 42 y.o. female admitted with sudden onset of slurred speech, right facial droop, and right UE and LE weakness. The patient's PMH includes the long-term use of birth control and HTN, which is uncontrolled. She has had a mild (R) CVA 1 year ago, but there are no residual impairments.

S: The patient states that she is having difficulty moving the (R) side of her body, the (R) UE more so than the (R) LE. She reports weakness in the right UE and LE.
PLOF: Independent with all functional mobility and ADLs without an assistive device. She worked full-time as a home health aide, drives, and takes care of her 12-year-old son. She is active in her child's activities and is also a volunteer in her community fire department. She is right-hand dominant.
Home Situation: She lives alone with her son in a split-entry home with 4-5 steps with a unilateral handrail to both the first and second levels of the home. Her parents do live close by and are supportive. They are in good health and are able to assist as needed.

O: *Swelling:* 3+ Pitting edema in right hand, decreased awareness of the right UE in general, and right facial droop with mild difficulty managing secretions.
Sensation: Impaired light touch, deep pressure, proprioception and kinesthesia to the right UE and LE but more so in the right UE.
Tone: The patient presents with decreased tone (hypotonia) with diminished reflexes 1+ throughout the right UE. Presents with increased extensor tone in the right LE, especially quadriceps, adductors, and plantarflexors. Modified Ashworth Scale[2] score for the right quads, adductors, and plantarflexors is 2.
MMT: Left UE and LE 5/5 throughout. Right UE: grossly 1/5 throughout all shoulder musculature, 0/5 elbow, forearm, hand, and wrist. Right LE: hip flexors 2/5, quadriceps 2+/5, abductors 1+/5, adductors 2+/5, hamstrings 2−/5, PF 2/5, DF 0/5.
Balance: Static sitting with close supervision depending on the compliance of the surface. Performs static standing with maximal assistance.
Modified Functional Reach Test[3]: Forward reach unaffected side was 17 cm; lateral reach to the left was 10 cm; lateral reach to the right (measure using acromion) was 2 cm.
Endurance: Able to tolerate and complete the 1-hour evaluation session with 1 rest break every 10-15 minutes. Her Borg Rating of Perceived Exertion following the examination was 12/20.
Functional Mobility
Bed Mobility: (L) Rolling: mod (A) x 1; (R) rolling min (a) x 1 and the use of the bed rail. Scooting: max (a) x 1. Supine to sit: max (a) x 1 for trunk control and safety.

Transfers: performs sit to stand from edge of bed with mod (A) x 1 with blocking of (R) knee to prevent buckling and for stabilization, postural control, and balance. Performs sit to stand out of w/c with maximal assistance and the same stabilization required, greater assistance required secondary to surface height difference. Bed to w/c transfers via stand pivot with moderate to maximal assistance of 1 depending on the surface height and direction in which transferring. Requires (R) knee to be blocked for stabilization and to prevent buckling.
Gait: The patient ambulated 20' along (L) handrail in hallway with max (a) x 1 and a close follow with the w/c. The patient required the (R) ankle to be ace wrapped into DF and slight eversion secondary to foot drop, decreased ankle control, and the inability to clear the foot during swing. The patient required manual assistance to complete swing, initiate the next step, and stabilize at the knee during stance to prevent buckling. She also required assistance for weight shifting to the right side and assistance at the pelvis to prevent pelvic retraction on the right.

A: The patient is a 42 y.o. female with the diagnosis of a (L) CVA with (R) hemiplegia. She has limited ROM and strength in the (R) UE and LE, limiting her basic functional mobility or ADLs without assistance. She is currently unable to care for herself or her son. Her prognosis is good for goals as stated and she would greatly benefit from inpatient acute rehabilitation for aggressive multidisciplinary services to meet her goals of returning home and therapy services to improve strength, balance, and functional mobility.

Problem List:

1. Edema in right UE
2. Decreased strength in right UE and LE
3. Impaired balance
4. Impaired bed mobility
5. Impaired transfers
6. Nonfunctional gait
7. Decreased endurance

STGs (to be met in 1 week):

1. The patient will verbalize and demonstrate understanding (R) UE awareness, positioning, and protection.
2. The patient will require min (a) x 1 for all bed mobility.
3. The patient will require mod (a) x 1 for all stand and squat pivot transfers to the right and left.
4. The patient will ambulate 50' with appropriate assistive device with mod (a) x 1 and minimal cueing for the (R) LE.
5. The patient will be (I) with static sitting.
6. Endurance will improve as evidence by tolerance to 1.5 to 2 hours of physical therapy daily for duration of stay.

LTGs (to be met in 3 weeks):

1. The patient will be independent with right UE management, care, and positioning.
2. The patient will demonstrate increased right UE and LE strength by at least 1 grade to help improve her ability to perform ADLs and mobility in the home.
3. The patient will be independent with all bed mobility.
4. The patient will require supervision for all transfers.
5. The patient will ambulate 150' with appropriate assistive device with supervision and the appropriate bracing if necessary.
6. The patient will be independent with static sitting balance and standing balance.
7. Her Modified Functional Reach score will improve more than 4 cm.
8. The patient will be able to return home with minimal assistance from caregivers.

P: The patient will be seen bid for 1.5 to 2 hours of physical therapy a day throughout duration of stay for neuromuscular re-education, strength, balance, and endurance training and functional mobility training. The patient will receive instruction on safe mobility, use of assistive device, and restoration of function. The patient will be provided with appropriate levels of assistance to assure safety. Treatment will be directed at meeting the stated goals with emphasis on increasing her function and ability to return home.

Note 1

One week later, you are working with the same 42-year-old woman who suffered a left CVA with right hemiplegia. Today, the case manager comes to you and informs you that an insurance update is needed and that the insurance is starting to question the need for continued inpatient acute rehabilitation. She wants a copy of your note for today's session. Review the documentation from the initial evaluation so that you are able to make the appropriate comparison to today's treatment for justification of continued need for skilled physical therapy services and acute rehabilitation. Try to summarize how the patient is progressing toward her goals as established by the PT, and write an appropriate plan that is consistent and within the above-stated plan of care.

Today, the patient expresses her excitement and pleasure at the rate at which she is progressing and has high hopes of returning home soon. Today, the patient required minimal assistance for all bed mobility and demonstrated the ability to incorporate the right UE into all tasks without the need for verbal reminders. Repetitive sit to stand and repetitive mat to wheelchair transfers via stand pivot performed for functional strength and endurance training with minimal assistance and only blocking of right knee 50% of the time secondary to fatigue. The patient ambulated 7' x 1 and 50' x 2 with a large-based quad cane with the right ankle ace wrapped into dorsiflexion with minimal assistance and manual assistance at the right LE for blocking and stabilization of the right knee during stance phase of gait to prevent buckling. The patient required rest breaks only between ambulation attempts for 1 to 2 minutes at a time. The patient continues to demonstrate right foot drop that likely requires a custom ankle-foot orthosis (AFO). She also continues to demonstrate weakness in the right upper and lower extremities evident by the need to manually block and stabilize the knee during transfers and gait as well as manual stabilization of the right UE secondary to weakness, especially during the sit to stand transition.

Note 2

After 3 weeks in acute inpatient rehabilitation, the patient demonstrates readiness for discharge to home with assistance from her family. The family is apprehensive and is in the clinic today for family training. Please document in SOAP format the family training session and the patient's and family's response to the training, and compare functional status findings from the previous note and the initial evaluation. Also, briefly comment on the status of her goals and write an appropriate plan.

The patient performed all bed mobility at a modified independence level and is independent in the care and positioning of her right UE. All transfers performed with supervision and verbal cues for safety. The patient is able to don her right AFO with minimal assistance and ambulated 150' with the large-based quad cane with supervision. The family was instructed in all functional mobility, proper guarding techniques, donning and doffing the AFO, assessing skin integrity, and wearing instructions. The family demonstrated competence both verbally and upon return demonstration with the ability to assist the patient in the home environment. The patient states that she is nervous about going home and expresses that she is still not independent with all functional mobility, which is where she would eventually like to be. She states that she would ultimately like to walk without an assistive device and no longer needs the assistance from her family.

Lower-Extremity Amputation/ Prosthetic Device

The following is an example of an initial evaluation written using an electronic documentation package for a patient recently admitted to a skilled nursing facility. Use it to help you complete the following 2 SOAP notes. Follow these directions as you write your notes:

- Write your notes to maximize reimbursement.
- Be specific when documenting your interventions (patient education, coordination or communication with other disciplines, and procedural intervention).
- Write your assessment and plan based on the information provided in the example and shown in the initial documentation that has been provided. Be sure to make comparisons between the patient's initial status and his current status.

PHYSICAL THERAPY INITIAL EXAMINATION

Patient's Name: John Hamilton

MR Number: #64591845A850

Date of Service: December 8, 2017

Date of Birth: January 15, 1944

PROBLEM: 73-year-old male 4 days s/p right transtibial amputation.

SUBJECTIVE

Pt. History: Long history of chronic wounds on the right foot; recently developed osteomyelitis and gangrene and underwent short transtibial amputation. Left elbow fracture 20 years ago.

Family History: Pt.'s mother had HTN and DM and his father had CAD.

Chief Complaint: Phantom pain from the left foot, poor mobility, and decreased endurance.

Current Pain Rating: 7/10

Worst Pain Rating: 9/10

Pain Characteristics: Aching, sharp, and burning pain in the residual limb; numbness around the suture line.

Prior Functional Status: Has never used an assistive device. Has been independent with all ADL and IADL prior to admission. Reports being active around his house and performing all home maintenance and yard work. Reports being an avid fisherman and participating in outdoor activities.

Living Situation: Pt. is retired Army sergeant. He lives alone in single-level house, with 2 steps at the entrance. Pt. 1 son living about 2 hours away who can assist on the weekends.

PMH: NIDDM, COPD, PVD, and HTN.

Health Habits: Pt. is a nonsmoker and nondrinker, although smoked 1 pack per day for 30 years. Quit when he was 50 y.o.

Pt.'s Goals: Return to independent, active life style, including driving. Wants to obtain a prosthetic device.

Communication: Pt. communicates goals and needs without difficulty.

OBJECTIVE

Vital Signs:

BP: 134/84

RR: 15

HR: 82

Palpation: Pulse at popliteal artery 2+ bilaterally.

Observation: Horizontal incision line at distal aspect of the residual limb, no tension, complete closure, no drainage.

AROM:

Upper Extremity:

	Right	**Left**
Shoulder flexion	160	160
Shoulder extension	45	45
Shoulder ER	90	90
Shoulder IR	70	70
Shoulder abduction	160	160
Shoulder adduction	0	0
Elbow	0/150	25/150
Wrist flexion	70	70
Wrist extension	70	70
Finger flexion	Full fist	Full fist
Finger extension	0	0

Lower Extremity:

	Right	**Left**
Hip flexion	90	140
Hip extension	0	20
Hip ER	45	45
Hip IR	10	10
Hip abduction	40	45
Hip adduction	0	0
Knee	10/90	0/150
Ankle PF	NA	50
Anke DF	NA	5

PROM:

Lower Extremity:

	Right	End Feel	Left	End Feel
Knee	5/110	Capsular	0	Normal

Strength:

Upper Extremity:

	Right	Left
Shoulder flexion	4/5	4/5
Shoulder extension	4/5	4/5
Shoulder ER	4/5	4/5
Shoulder IR	4/5	4/5
Shoulder abduction	4/5	4/5
Shoulder adduction	4/5	4/5
Elbow	4/5	4/5
Wrist flexion	4/5	4/5
Wrist extension	4/5	4/5
Finger flexion	4/5	4/5
Finger extension	4/5	4/5

Lower Extremity:

	Right	Left
Hip flexion	Not assessed due to surgery	4/5
Hip extension	Not assessed due to surgery	4/5
Hip ER	Not assessed due to surgery	4/5
Hip IR	Not assessed due to surgery	4/5
Hip abduction	Not assessed due to surgery	4/5
Hip adduction	Not assessed due to surgery	4/5
Knee	Not assessed due to surgery	4/5
Ankle PF	NA	4/5
Ankle DF	NA	4/5

Anthropometric Measurements:

Girth	Right	Left
Knee joint	38 cm	35 cm
2" below	37 cm	35 cm
4" below	37 cm	35 cm

Other: Residual limb length: 4' from tibial tuberosity

Sensation: Left LE is intact to light touch; right residual limb demonstrates diminished light touch sensation around suture line.

Balance:

Static Sitting: Normal

Static Standing: Decreased

Dynamic Sitting: Normal

Dynamic Standing: Decreased

Modified Functional Reach Test: Forward 30 cm, Right 12 cm, Left 15 cm

Functional Reach Test: 5 cm (performed with close supervision)

Mobility:

Wheelchair Mobility: Max assist x 1 for parts management and propels 20' with verbal cues on level surfaces.

Bed Mobility:

Rolling: Independent

Scooting: Independent

Bridging: Independent

Supine to Sit: Min assist x 1

Sit to Supine: Min assist x 1

Transfers:

Sit to Stand: Min assist x 1

Stand to Sit: Min assist x 1

Bed to Chair: Min assist x 1

Chair to Bed: Min assist x 1

Toilet: Min assist x 1

Floor: Not assessed

Gait:

Parallel Bars: 10' with CGA x 1

Even Surface: 25' with standard walker requiring min (A) x 1 for sequencing and balance.

Uneven Surface: Not assessed

Treatment:

Treatment	Side	Prescription
Ther ex: hip flexion	Bilateral	2 x 10 to increase ROM
Ther ex: hip extension	Bilateral	2 x 10 to increase ROM
Ther ex: hip abduction	Bilateral	2 x 10 to increase ROM
Ther ex: hip adduction	Bilateral	2 x 10 to increase ROM
Ther ex: knee flexion	Bilateral	2 x 10 to increase ROM
Ther ex: knee extension	Bilateral	2 x 10 to increase ROM
Ther ex: hamstring stretching	Right	3 x 30 seconds to increase knee extension
Ther ex: other: towel propping	Right	5 minutes to increase knee extension
Pt. ed: towel propping	Right	To be done 5 minutes tid
Initial evaluation		
Treatment time		60 minutes

PLAN OF CARE

Assessment: Impaired ROM, gait, locomotion, and balance associated with amputation limiting pt.'s ability to return home to independent, safe living.

Prognosis: Good

Barriers to Treatment: Comorbidities

Need for Skilled Services: Pt. requiring skilled services for improving functional mobility including gait and transfer training with assistive devices due to amputation. Also required for preparing residual limb for prosthesis, improving joint mobility needed for prosthetic gait, education on skin integrity, gait training, and safe progression of mobility once he obtains the prosthetic device.

Problem List

Impairments:

1. A/PROM right LE; especially hip flexion, extension, and knee extension
2. Decreased strength right LE
3. Decreased sensation
4. Edema
5. Incision present
6. Impaired balance
7. Phantom pain (7/10)
8. Decreased endurance

Activity Limitations/Participation Restrictions:

1. Decreased independence with bed mobility
2. Decreased independence with transfers
3. Decreased independence with ambulation
4. Decreased independence with wheelchair mobility
5. Unable to perform home management tasks
6. Unable to drive
7. Unable to perform necessary IADL (eg, grocery shopping, going to bank)
8. Unable to participate in usual lifestyle

Anticipated Goals and Expected Outcomes

Pt./family will:

1. Demonstrate full A/PROM in the right LE with no contractures—necessary for normal prosthetic ambulation in 8 weeks.
2. Achieve right LE strength to 4/5 also to allow normal prosthetic ambulation in 8 weeks.
3. Be independent with skin care and monitoring skin with use of prosthesis in 8 weeks.
4. Decrease residual limb edema 100% compared to opposite side to prepare for prosthetic device.
5. Demonstrate 100% healing of his incision in 8 weeks.
6. Report a 50% reduction in c/o phantom pain in 8 weeks.
7. Be independent with all bed mobility in 8 weeks.
8. Perform sit to and from stand independently in 8 weeks.
9. Ambulate 500' with walker independently to allow home and limited community mobility in 8 weeks.
10. Ambulate 250' independently with prosthesis and least restrictive assistive device in 8 weeks.
11. Manage wheelchair parts and propel wheelchair for unlimited distances independently in 8 weeks.
12. Participate in driving assessment to identify car modifications in 8 weeks.

Treatment Plan:
See pt. for 1 hour bid daily for 8 weeks to work on the above through active and passive exercise, endurance training, gait (including prosthetic) and transfer training, pain modulation to decrease phantom pain, balance, and pt. education. Will also work on edema control. Pt. is motivated and agrees with the above plan.

Therapist:
Betty Smith, PT

Date/Time of electronic signature: 12/8/17 15:35

License Number #4444

____________________________ ________________________

Physician Signature Date

Note 1

The patient is now 2 weeks status post right transtibial amputation. He is continuing to complain of phantom pain (current pain rating, 6/10) and sensation from the right foot. It resolves if he "squeezes" his residual limb. You are planning to attend a team conference for him on the following day, so you decide to take some objective measurements. Right AROM: Hip flexion 120°, extension 5°, abduction 40°, adduction 10°, knee flexion 130°, knee extension -5°. PROM: Right knee extension 0°. Strength: Right LE hip flexion 4/5, extension holds against moderate resistance in side lying position, abduction holds against moderate resistance in side lying position, knee extension holds against minimal resistance in seated position, knee flexion holds against moderate resistance in side lying position. The patient cannot lie prone due to pulmonary problems and difficulty breathing when in this position. The incision is healing well. There is no drainage and no s/s of infection. It is moderately adhered to the underlying tissue and hypersensitive to pressure. Residual Limb Girth: 36.2 cm at the knee joint, 35 cm 2" below, and 35 cm 4" below. The patient can move and transfer in and out of bed independently to a bedside commode or chair. He can manage the wheelchair parts with verbal cueing. He propels the wheelchair 50' independently on level surfaces and carpet and then requires a rest. He can ambulate 75' with a standard walker with supervision x 1 and good balance.

You spend the next 30 minutes on therapeutic exercise to improve AROM and PROM in the residual limb, strength in the sound limb and upper extremities, and balance. You spend 30 minutes on gait and transfer training. You will discuss prosthetic options with the physical therapist and, if appropriate, with the rehabilitation team the following day.

Note 2

The patient is now 8 weeks s/p right transtibial amputation. He is continuing to complain of phantom pain (2/10) and sensation from the right foot occasionally, but it has decreased by about 75%. He has had a temporary prosthesis for about 2 days. Right AROM is as follows: Hip flexion 120°, extension 10°, abduction 40°, adduction 10°, knee flexion 130°, knee extension 0°. Strength: Right LE hip flexion 4/5, extension holds against moderate resistance in side lying position, abduction holds against moderate resistance in side lying position, knee extension holds against moderate resistance in seated position, knee flexion holds against maximum resistance in side lying position. The incision is not adhered to the underlying tissue and sensitivity has subsided approximately 50%. Residual Limb Girth: 35 cm at the knee joint, 35 cm 2" below, and 35 cm 4" below. He is independent with all wheelchair parts and transfers. He propels the wheelchair 500' independently on level surfaces and carpet. He can ambulate 150' with axillary crutches with supervision x 1 and good balance without the prosthesis. You spend 30 minutes on prosthetic training. He requires minimal assistance to don and doff the socket. He ambulates 50' with the prosthesis on and with axillary crutches with minimal assistance for weight shifting. He is ambulating with an abducted gait on the prosthetic side. You spend 10 minutes educating the patient on skin precautions after removing the prosthesis and 30 minutes on exercises, including passive stretching for the right hip flexors and hamstrings, strengthening for the residual limb, endurance, and balance. You spend 15 minutes on gait training.

Musculoskeletal Trauma

The following is an example of an initial evaluation written using an electronic documentation package for a patient recently seen in an outpatient clinic. Use it to help you complete the following 2 SOAP notes. Follow these directions as you write your notes:

- Write your notes to maximize reimbursement.
- Be specific when documenting your interventions (include patient education, coordination or communication with other disciplines, and procedural intervention).
- Write your assessment and plan based on the information provided in the example and shown in the initial documentation that has been provided. Be sure to make comparisons between the patient's initial status and his current status.

ANYTOWN PHYSICAL THERAPY

1111 West Midtown Road

Baltimore, MD 12345

(555) 111-2345

Patient: Michael T. Smith

DOB: 3/5/1989

Date: September, 1 2017

MRN: 49845V94KED

Physician: Jay Brown, MD

PHYSICAL THERAPY EXAMINATION

Reason for Referral: 28 y.o. male s/p left wrist and ankle fracture referred to physical therapy to begin gentle wrist and ankle AROM and PROM and to begin using crutches with a platform for the left UE; pt. is PWB 50% on left LE.

Diagnosis: Left distal radius fracture; left tibia-fibula fracture.

Date of Injury: 8/1/16

History: 4 weeks s/p fall (~25") from a logging truck landing on his left side. Pt. sustained fracture of the left distal radius and ulna and left distal tibia and fibula. Pt. underwent ORIF for the wrist and ankle immediately after the injury. He was placed in a short-arm cast for the UE and short-leg cast for the LE. He was non-weightbearing on the left LE and has been unable to use crutches because he has not been allowed to bear weight on the affected UE. At the time of the fall, pt. also sustained a mild concussion. He was hospitalized for 5 days following the injury. While hospitalized, he received inpatient therapy to learn how to negotiate his wheelchair and to perform transfers. The arm cast was removed 2 weeks ago and he was placed into a removable wrist orthosis that he wore at all times. The leg cast was removed yesterday and his ankle was placed in a removable orthosis.

Chief Complaint: Pain and stiffness in left UE and LE with decreased functional use of both. Doesn't like using wheelchair for mobility. Unable to work. Requiring assistance with self-care activities and home management.

Current Pain Level: 2/10

Worst Pain Level: 1/10

Pain Area: Left wrist; left ankle

Pain Behavior: Aching, intermittent, daytime, decreasing

PMH: No significant medical history

Medication(s): Ibuprofen PRN

Social Situation: Right-hand dominant; lives with wife and 2 small children in single-level home with 2 steps at entrance with a handrail on the right. Prior to injury, pt. was employed by logging company and also worked as a contractor. He has been off work since the date of injury. Pt. is unable to drive and is relying on his wife and mother for transportation. No significant prior medical history or history of fracture. Reports being a nonsmoker and nondrinker. Family history is positive for OA.

Functional Status:

Function	Current	Prior	Patient Goal
Ambulation	Unable to perform	Independent	Yes
Stairs	Unable to perform	Independent	Yes
ADLs and self-care	Needs assist	Independent	Yes
Home management	Unable to perform	Independent	Yes
Driving	Unable to perform	Independent	Yes
Work	Unable to perform	Independent	Yes

Functional Measures:

DASH[4]	78/100
FAAM[5] (ADL subscale)	4/84

Observation:

Healed suture lines on the volar aspect of the left wrist and the medial and lateral aspect of the left lower leg. Scars are pink and slightly raised. No s/s of infection.

Girth:

	Right	Left
Wrist figure 8	36 cm	37.2 cm
Ankle figure 8	42 cm	44.1 cm

Hand — AROM:

	Right	Left
Finger flexion	WNL	WNL
Finger extension	WNL	WNL
Comments: Able to close his fingers into a tight full fist and open without limitations; opposes the thumb to the distal palmar crease.		

Wrist — AROM:

	Right	Left
Wrist flexion	90	20
Wrist extension	90	10
Radial deviation	20	10
Ulnar deviation	30	5
Forearm supination	80	30
Forearm pronation	80	40
Comments: Elbow and shoulder AROM are WNL bilateral.		

Ankle — AROM:

	Right	**Left**
Ankle dorsiflexion	5	-10
Ankle plantarflexion	50	25
Ankle inversion	50	15
Ankle eversion	5	0
Comments: Knee and Hip AROM are WNL bilateral.		

Wrist — PROM:

	Right	**Left**
Wrist flexion	30	Empty
Wrist extension	20	Empty
Radial deviation	10	Empty
Ulnar deviation	5	Empty
Forearm supination	35	Empty
Forearm pronation	45	Empty

Ankle — PROM:

	Right	**Left**
Ankle dorsiflexion	-5	Empty
Ankle plantarflexion	30	Empty
Ankle inversion	25	Empty
Ankle eversion	0	Empty
Comments: Knee and Hip AROM are WNL bilateral.		

Wrist — Strength:

	Right	**Left**
Wrist flexion	5/5	2-/5
Wrist extension	5/5	2-/5
Radial deviation	5/5	2-/5
Ulnar deviation	5/5	2-/5
Forearm supination	5/5	2-/5
Forearm pronation	5/5	2-/5

Ankle — Strength:

	Right	Left
Wrist flexion	5/5	2-/5
Wrist extension	5/5	2-/5
Radial deviation	5/5	2-/5
Ulnar deviation	5/5	2-/5
Forearm supination	5/5	2-/5
Forearm pronation	5/5	2-/5

Sensation:

	Right	Left
Common peroneal	Intact to light touch	Intact to light touch
Saphenous	Intact to light touch	Intact to light touch
Superficial peroneal	Intact to light touch	Intact to light touch
Deep peroneal	Intact to light touch	Intact to light touch
Medial plantar	Intact to light touch	Intact to light touch
Lateral plantar	Intact to light touch	Intact to light touch
Radial	Intact to light touch	Intact to light touch
Median	Intact to light touch	Intact to light touch
Ulnar	Intact to light touch	Intact to light touch

Palpation: Tenderness at the scars; scars are adhered to the underlying skin; 2+ at radial and dorsal pedal arteries on the left; intact capillary refill on the right hand and foot.

Functional Assessment:

	Performance
Supine to/from sit	Independent
Sit to/from stand	Independent
Gait	Ambulated with axillary crutches with platform for left UE. He was PWB 50% left LE using step to gait pattern. Pt. required contact guard assist x 1 for balance and for managing the left crutch/platform.
Stairs	Deferred at this time

Plan of Care:

Assessment: 28 y.o. RHD male 4 wks s/p fall where he sustained left wrist and ankle fractures. Underwent surgery 4 weeks ago for both but is now presenting with impaired strength and ROM limiting function in the left wrist and ankle including limiting self-care, ambulation, home management, work, and recreational activities. Pt. demonstrates excellent motivation and good potential for full recovery. No comorbidities that could affect outcome identified at this time.

Problems:

1. Decreased AROM in the left wrist and ankle limiting ADLs, self-care, and work activities
2. Decreased strength in the left wrist and ankle limiting ADLs, self-care, and work activities
3. Increased edema in the left wrist and ankle limiting AROM
4. Adhering scars on the left wrist and ankle limiting AROM
5. Decreased independence with gait
6. Unable to perform independent ADLs
7. Unable to perform independent home management
8. Unable to perform independent self-care
9. Unable to drive
10. Unable to work

Short-Term Goals To Be Met By: 10/1/17

At the end of 2 weeks, pt. will:

1. Increase AROM 10°–15° for the wrist, forearm, and ankle to allow normal functional activities.
2. Decrease edema by 0.5 cm for the wrist and ankle to allow increased ROM.
3. Ambulate with crutches with UE platform independently for 1000 feet.
4. Perform all self-care independently.
5. Decrease DASH Score by > 15%.
6. Improve FAAM score by > 10%.

Long-Term Goals To Be Met By: 1/1/18

At the end of 16 weeks (d/c), pt. will:

1. Have AROM of the wrist, forearm, and ankle 90% to 100% of opposite to allow normal use during ADL, home management, and work activities.
2. Grip and pinch strength will be 80% to 100% of right to allow normal use during ADL, home management, and work activities.
3. Be independent with all home management tasks.
4. Ambulate independently on all surfaces without the use of an assistive device.
5. Ascend and descend a flight of stairs independently without the use of an assistive device.
6. Drive without restrictions.
7. RTW at previous level of employment.
8. DASH Score < 20.
9. FAAM ADL Score > 70.

Plan: See pt. 3x/wk for next 3-4 mos. to work on AROM and PROM of the wrist and ankle; general LE ex. for the hip, knee, shoulder, and elbow; gait training; functional mobility; and strengthening when appropriate. Will progress pt. as tolerated and according to MD orders. Skilled services will be provided to instruct patient in appropriate ther ex and progression, use of assistive device, and progression of gait as ordered. Pt. will also require strengthening and functional mobility retraining to prepare for return to normal living situation and RTW. Pt. is in agreement with the above-stated plan.

Initial Treatment:

Service	Details	Time
Initial examination		30 minutes
Therapeutic – exercise – hand	AROM left wrist for flexion, extension, supination	15 minutes
	PROM left wrist for flexion, extension, supination	
Therapeutic – exercise – ankle	AROM and PROM left ankle DF and PF, used opposite foot for self PROM of ankle	15 minutes
Gait training	As above	15 minutes
Patient education	HEP as shown above	
	Weightbearing restriction	
	Use of crutches	
	Use of compression with wrap for edema control	

John Smith, PT
Electronically signed 9/1/17 14:55

Note 1

The patient is now 6 weeks s/p fall (has received 2 weeks of outpatient therapy). He is reporting improvement in his ability to perform self-care, achieve a full fist, and ambulate. He thinks the exercises are helping to improve all of these activities. He is seeing the doctor today and is hoping to be able to discontinue the use of the crutches. You take the following AROM measurements for the left wrist: flexion 50°, extension 35°, supination 50°, pronation 60°, left ankle 0° and 45° of PF. He has 10° of inversion and 2° of eversion. He can perform all transfers independently and ambulates 100' independently PWB (50%) on the left LE with crutches with a left platform. Wrist figure 8 is 36.7 cm on the left and ankle figure 8 is 43.4 on the left. You are still not performing strength assessment due to fractures. You spend 45 minutes working on exercises to increase ROM for the ankle and wrist and reviewing his home exercises. DASH score is 55 and FAAM score is 21.

Note 2

The patient is now 9 weeks s/p fall. He is reporting independence with self-care, ambulation, and driving. He thinks that the exercises are helping to improve all of these activities and to improve strength necessary for returning to work. He is ambulating full weight bearing on the left, without the use of crutches. You take the following AROM measurements for the left wrist: flexion 80°, extension 75°, supination 75°, pronation 80°, left ankle 5° DF, and has 50° of PF. He has 15° of inversion and 5° of eversion. He can ambulate for unlimited distances around the house and the community. He does have some mild swelling after ambulating distances greater than 400' to 500'. Wrist figure 8 is 36 cm on the left and ankle figure 8 is 43 on the left. Grip strength measured via grip dynamometer (#2 handle spacing) was 120 pounds on the right and 62 pounds on the left. You spend 45 minutes working on exercises to increase ROM and for the ankle and wrist, and reviewing his home exercises. DASH score is 44 and FAAM is 68.

Pediatric/Orthotic Devices

The following is an example of an initial evaluation written using an electronic documentation package for a patient recently seen in an outpatient clinic. Use it to help you complete the following 2 SOAP notes. Follow these directions as you write your notes:

- Write your notes to maximize reimbursement.
- Be specific when documenting your interventions (include patient education, coordination or communication with other disciplines, and procedural intervention).
- Write your assessment and plan based on the information provided in the example and shown in the initial documentation that has been provided. Be sure to make comparisons between the patient's initial status and his current status.

Pediatric Case

Pr: 5-year-old girl with L3 level myelomeningocele, referred to PT for transfer training, gait training, and KAFO management.

S: *Hx*: Myelomeningocele present at birth. Immediate surgery to repair. Resultant L3 incomplete paralysis. No history of hydrocephalus or seizure disorder.
C/C: Impaired ability to transfer independently; decreased independence with ambulation.
L/S: Lives with both parents, who are very supportive. Attends kindergarten at a local, public elementary school.
Pt.'s and Parents' goals: Increase independence with transfers, participate in circle time on the floor without having to be transferred by the teacher, ambulate household distances and short distances while at school independently, manage wheelchair independently.
Cognition/Communication: Able to communicate without difficulty and expresses goals of therapy. At grade level for all school-related cognitive tasks per parental report.

O: *AROM*: Both UEs are WNL; LEs: (B) hip flexion 120°, extension 0°, abduction 20°, adduction 10°; knee flexion 50°, knee extension 0°.
PROM: Bilateral hip extension 20°, hip abduction 45°, knees 0°-135°; ankle DF 20° and PF 50°.
Strength: Both UEs 4/5 throughout; LEs: (R) hip flexion 3+/5, hip extension 2-/5, hip abduction 2-/5, hip adduction 3+/5; knee extension 3/5, knee flexion 2-/5; (L) hip flexion 4/5, hip extension 2-/5; hip abduction 2-/5, hip adduction 4/5; knee extension 3+/5, knee flexion 2-/5.
Sensation: (R): Normal sensation in L1 and 2; diminished in L3, L4, and L5; absent in S1. (L): Normal sensation in L1, 2, and 3 dermatomes; diminished light touch in L4 and L5; absent in S1.
Posture: Normal spinal alignment and absence of joint contractures or abnormal posture of feet and ankles.
Spasticity: Mild in both hip adductors and heel cords right > left. Modified Ashworth Scale[2] (R) 2, (L) 1+.
Bowel/Bladder: Incontinent in bowel and bladder control but is independently managed by parents and teacher.
Skin Condition: No impairments other than small area on right navicular from pressure from orthotic device.

Anthropometrics: Normal body weight for height.
Balance: Not impaired when standing in parallel bars with bilateral UE support.
Bed Mobility: Independent rolling and scooting.
Transfers: Supine to and from long and short sit independently; sit to and from stand with minimal assist x 1 using Lofstrand crutches and KAFOs; w/c to and from floor with supervision.
Floor Mobility: Independent in floor mobility for short distances using commando crawling.
Wheelchair Management/Mobility: Independent with mobility on level even surfaces for 50-60'; requires minimal assist x 1 for managing parts including leg rests and arm rests.
Gait: Ambulated 10' x 1 with minimal assist x 1 using step to gait with KAFO knees locked at 0°. Balance impaired when ambulating with Lofstrands due to decreased proprioception and kinesthetic awareness of both LEs.
Endurance: Unable to ambulate more than 10' without shortness of breath.
Orthotic Devices: Dependent in donning and doffing.

A: 5-year-old girl presents with impaired motor function and sensory integrity associated with nonprogressive disorder of the CNS. Prognosis for anticipated goals and outcomes is good. Skilled services needed to educate and train patient and family members on appropriate ways to transfer, for endurance and strengthening to promote increased independence with gait and transfers.

Problem List:

1. Bilateral LE weakness
2. Flaccid ankles
3. Impaired proprioception and kinesthetic awareness during gait
4. Impaired sensation
5. Mild spasticity
6. Impaired endurance
7. Decreased ability to transfer from wheelchair to floor
8. Decreased independence with sit to and from stand
9. Decreased independence with gait
10. Decreased ability to safely ambulate functional distances at home and at school
11. Requires assistance for managing wheelchair parts
12. Requires assistance to manage orthotic devices

Anticipated goals and expected outcomes: At the end of 8 weeks, pt. will:

1. Transfer w/c to and from floor with minimal assist x 1
2. Perform sit to and from stand independently
3. Manage wheelchair leg rests and arm rests independently
4. Propel w/c 500' independently
5. Ambulate 100' with knee ankle foot orthoses (KAFOs) and bilateral
6. Lofstrand crutches with close supervision
7. Don and doff the KAFOs with minimal assistance

P: See pt. 2-3 x per week to work on the above plan and goals. Will require strengthening, endurance, balance, and gait training to meet above goals. Pt. and parent are in agreement with above plan.

Note 1

It is now the patient's fourth physical therapist visit, and you have been working with this patient for the last 2 visits. She is very motivated and happy to come to therapy. She is very cooperative and her parents are very supportive and follow through with all instructions as assigned. She demonstrates the ability to transfer from the wheelchair to the floor with minimal assistance and verbal cueing. She requires moderate assistance to transfer from the floor to the wheelchair. Her UE strength is good via manual muscle test, but she cannot lift her own body weight at this point. She performs sit to and from stand with contact guard assistance with the KAFOs and Lofstrand crutches. She can ambulate 40' with minimal assistance of 1 with the braces and crutches also. She is still demonstrating impaired dynamic balance. You work with her for 30 minutes performing UE and LE strengthening and dynamic balance exercises and for an additional 15 minutes on gait training.

Note 2

The patient has been participating in physical therapist for 1 month, you have seen her at every visit with the exceptions of the initial evaluation and during a reevaluation that took place approximately 1 to 2 weeks ago. She is still very cooperative and motivated. She received new KAFOs from the orthotist today. They have a manual locking mechanism at the knee and are rigid at the ankles. Inspection of the devices reveals no problems with hardware, and all edges and rivets are smooth and straps are well secured. The skin is free from breakdown before donning the devices. The patient requires moderate assistance to don the orthotic devices and to engage the knee lock. She ambulates in the parallel bars 10' using an open-hand technique with minimal assistance of 1 and then uses her Lofstrands using a step to gait pattern also requiring minimal assist. After gait training (lasted approximately 20 minutes) the patient requires moderate assistance to doff the orthotic devices. The patient and parents are educated on skin inspection. There was a small area on the right navicular that was red after removing the device on the right. You provide education on monitoring the redness. Leaving the braces off, you perform 30 minutes of exercises for the UEs and LEs and dynamic balance activities.

Documentation Practice 1

You are working with a patient with a diagnosis of left bicipital tendinitis in an outpatient clinic. She tells you that she has been working on the home exercises and that, overall, her arm is feeling much better. She reports pain to be 3/10 on a verbal pain scale. She says that she has trouble reaching into overhead cabinets and shelves. Her AROM at the left shoulder is 124° flexion, 110° abduction, 50° external rotation, and 35° internal rotation. Her treatment consists of ultrasound over the anterior shoulder for 6 minutes, 50% duty cycle, with the intensity set at 1.5 w/cm^2. This is followed by gentle AROM exercises with a wand for flexion and external rotation, active scapular retraction and protraction, prone horizontal abduction, and external rotation with yellow exercise band for 2 sets of 10 repetitions. She also receives manual stretching for flexion, internal rotation, and external rotation (performed by you). The treatment concludes with ice for 15 minutes. She reports better ROM and less pain (1/10) when the treatment is over. You measure active motion post-treatment and flexion as 145°, abduction as 125°, external rotation as 65°, and internal rotation as 50°. She will return 2 times each week for the above treatment and progression of the exercises as tolerated.

Documentation Practice 2

You are working with a patient 3 days status post-right total knee replacement in the physical therapy gym. She rates her pain as a 6/10. She tells you that she is going to a skilled nursing facility later in the week. Her AROM in the knee is 10/55°. She has noticeable swelling and limited ROM in the knee and ankle. She transfers to and from the mat with you providing 25% assistance. She transfers sit to and from supine with you performing 50% assistance due to her inability to lift the right leg onto the mat table. She performs 2 sets of 10 repetitions of the total knee exercises and ambulates 50 feet, twice, with a standard walker, only putting 50% of her body weight on the involved extremity. Her active knee motion after treatment is 5/75°. She receives ice for 15 minutes to her knee. You notice that she walked only 25' during yesterday's session and that her transfers required moderate assistance. She will be seen in the afternoon for the same treatment, progressing gait as tolerated.

References

1. *About the FIM System®*. Uniform Data System for Medical Rehabilitation website. https://www.udsmr.org/WebModules/FIM/Fim_About.aspx. Accessed July 16, 2017.
2. Bohannon RW, Smith MB. Interrater reliability of a modified Ashworth scale of muscle spasticity. *Phys Ther.* 1987;67(2):206-207.
3. Katz-Leurer M, Fisher I, Neeb M, Scwartz I, Carmeli E. Reliability and validity of the modified functional reach test at the sub-acute stage post-stroke. *Disabil Rehabil.* 2009;31(3):243-248.
4. Hudak PL, Amadio PC, Bombardier C. Development of an upper extremity outcome measure: the DASH (disabilities of the arm, shoulder and hand) [corrected]. The Upper Extremity Collaborative Group (UECG). *Am J Ind Med.* 1996;29(6):602-608.
5. Martin RL, Irrgang JJ, Burdett RG, Conti SF, Van Swearingen JM. Evidence of validity for the Foot and Ankle Ability Measure (FAAM). *Foot Ankle Int.* 2005;26(11):968-983.

Appendix

Abbreviations and Symbols

This list provides many of the abbreviations and symbols used in medical charts and in physical therapy records. Because documentation styles can vary, you should check with your facility regarding abbreviations and symbols that are "approved" for use. Also, note that some abbreviations have more than one meaning. Be sure to understand the context in which each abbreviation is used. Lists are alphabetized by the abbreviation.

Abbreviations

A: or "**A**": assessment
a, (a), or **(A)**: assist (min, mod, max)
AAROM: active assistive range of motion
Ab: antibody
abd: abduction
ABG(s): arterial blood gas(es)
ac: before meals
ACE: angiotensin-converting enzyme
Ach: acetylcholine
ACL: anterior cruciate ligament
ad lib: as desired
AD: assistive device; Alzheimer's disease
ADA: Americans with Disabilities Act
add: adduction
ADL: activities of daily living
ADM: abductor digiti minimi
AE: above elbow
AFB: acid-fast bacilli
AFO: ankle-foot orthosis
AGA: appropriate for gestational age
AIDS: acquired immunodeficiency syndrome
AK: above knee
AKA: above-knee amputation
ALL: acute lymphoblastic leukemia
ALS: amyotrophic lateral sclerosis
am: before noon
AMA: against medical advice
AMB or **amb**: ambulatory
AML: acute myeloblastic leukemia
ANOVA: analysis of variance
AP: ankle pump; anterior-posterior
APB: abductor pollicus brevis
APL: abductor pollicus longus
ARDS: adult (acute) respiratory distress syndrome
AROM: active range of motion
ASA: aspirin
ASAP: as soon as possible
ASHD: arteriosclerotic heart disease
ATF: anterior talofibular
AV: atriovenous

B, (B), bil: both or bilateral
BBB: blood-brain barrier
BE: below elbow
bid: twice daily
BK: below knee
BKA: below-knee amputation
BLE or **(B)LE**: bilateral lower extremities
BM: bowel movement
BMD: bone mineral density
BMI: body mass index
BP: blood pressure

Erickson ML, McKnight R. *Documentation Basics for the Physical Therapist Assistant, Third Edition* (pp. 155-160)

BPH: benign prostatic hypertrophy
BPM or **bpm**: beats per minute
BRP: bathroom privileges
BSA: body surface area
BSC: bedside commode
BUN: blood urea nitrogen

C & S: culture and sensitivity
Ca: calcium
CA: cancer
CABG: coronary artery bypass graft
CAD: coronary artery disease
CAT: computerized axial tomography
CBC: complete blood count
c/c or **C/C**: chief complaint
cc or **cm3**: cubic centimeter
CCU: critical (or coronary) care unit
CDC: Centers for Disease Control
CF: calcaneofibular
CF: cystic fibrosis
CGA: contact guard assist
CHI: closed head injury
CHO: carbohydrate
Cl: chlorine
cm: centimeter
CMC: carpometacarpal
CMS: Centers for Medicare & Medicaid Services
CMV: cytomegalovirus
CNS: central nervous system
c/o: complains of
COPD: chronic obstructive pulmonary disease
CORF: comprehensive outpatient rehabilitation facility
COTA: certified occupational therapist assistant
CP: cerebral palsy
CPAP: continuous positive airway pressure
CPM: continuous passive motion
CPR: cardiopulmonary resuscitation
CSF: cerebrospinal fluid
CT: computed tomography
CV: cardiovascular
CVA: cerebrovascular accident
CWP: cold whirlpool
cx: cancel; crutches

(D): dependent
DASH: Disabilities of the Arm, Shoulder and Hand disability questionnaire
DC: doctor of chiropractic; chiropractor
d/c: discharge or discontinue
DF: dorsiflexion
DI: dorsal interossei
DIP: distal interphalangeal
DJD: degenerative joint disease
DM: diabetes mellitus
DME: durable medical equipment
DO: doctor of osteopath
DOI: date of injury
DRG: diagnosis-related group
DRUJ: distal radioulnar joint
DTR: deep tendon reflex
DVT: deep vein thrombosis
dx: diagnosis

ea.: each
ECF: extracellular fluid
ECRB: extensor carpi radialis brevis
ECRL: extensor carpi radialis longus
ECU: extensor carpi ulnaris
EDC: extensor digitorum communis
EDM: extensor digiti minimi
EEG: electroencephalogram
EENT: eyes, ears, nose, and throat
EIP: extensor indicis proprius
EKG, ECG: electrocardiogram
EMG: electromyogram
EMS: emergency medical services
ENG: electronystagmograph
EO: elbow orthosis
EOB: edge of bed
EPB: extensor pollicus brevis
EPL: extensor pollicus longus
ERV: expiratory reserve volume
ESR: erythrocyte sedimentation rate
ESRD: end-stage renal disease
EtOH or **ETOH**: ethyl alcohol
ev, ever: eversion
ex.: exercise

F or **3/5**: fair (manual muscle test)
FBS: fasting blood sugar
FCR: flexor carpi radialis
FCU: flexor carpi ulnaris
FDA: Food and Drug Administration
FDM: flexor digiti minimi
FDP: flexor digitorum profundus
FDS: flexor digitorum superficialis
FES: functional electrical stimulation
FEV: forced expiratory volume
FHR: fetal heart rate
fl: fluid
FM: fibromyalgia syndrome
FO: foot orthosis
FPB: flexor pollicus brevis
FPL: flexor pollicus longus
FRC: functional residual capacity
FTSG: full thickness skin graft
FUO: fever of unknown origin
FVC: forced vital capacity
FWB: full weightbearing
FWW: front-wheeled walker
fx: fracture

G or 4/5: good (manual muscle test)
g: gram
GA: gestational age
GERD: gastroesophageal reflux disease
GH: glenohumeral
GI: gastrointestinal
GS: gluteal sets
GTT: glucose tolerance test

H & H: hemoglobin and hematocrit
H & P: history and physical
h or hr: hour
H_2O: water
HAV: hepatitis A virus; hallux abductovalgus
Hb: hemoglobin
HBV: hepatitis B virus
HCFA: Health Care Financing Administration
HCPCS: health care common procedure coding system
Hct: hematocrit
HCV: hepatitis C virus
HDL: high-density lipoprotein
HEP: home exercise program
HHA: home health agency
HIV: human immunodeficiency virus
HMO: health maintenance organization
HNP: herniated nucleus pulposus
h/o: history of
HO: hand orthosis
HO: hip orthosis
HOB: head of bed
HP: hot pack
HPI: history of present illness
HR: handrail; heart rate
HRT: hormone replacement therapy
HTN: hypertension
hx: history
Hz: hertz

(I): independent
I & D: incision and drainage
I & O: intake and output
IADL: instrumental activities of daily living
IC: inspiratory capacity
ICD: International Classification of Diseases
ICF: intracellular fluid; *International Classification of Functioning, Disability and Health*
ICIDH: *International Classification of Impairments, Disabilities, and Handicaps*
ICP: intracranial pressure
ICU: intensive care unit
IDDM: insulin-dependent diabetes mellitus
IDEA: Individuals with Disabilities in Education Act
Ig: immunoglobulin
IM: intramuscular
INH: isoniazid
inv: inversion
IP: inpatient; interphalangeal
IPPS: inpatient prospective payment system
IRV: inspiratory reserve volume
IV: intravenous

K: potassium
KAFO: knee-ankle-foot orthosis
kg: kilogram

L: liter
L or (L): left
LAC: long-arm cast
LAQ: long arc quadriceps exercise
LB: lower body
LBQC: large-base quad cane
LCL: lateral collateral ligament
LDL: low-density lipoprotein
LE: lower extremity
LHD: left-hand dominant
LLC: long-leg cast
LMN: lower motor neuron
LMRP: local medical review policies
LP: lumbar puncture
L/S, l/s: lifestyle
LT: lunotriquetrial
LTFG: long-term functional goal
LTG: long-term goal
LTM: long-term memory

m: meter
m.: muscle
MAS: Modified Ashworth Scale
max: maximum
MCA: motorcycle accident
MCL: medial collateral ligament
MCP: metacarpophalangeal
MD: muscular dystrophy; medical doctor/physician
MED(s): medicines, medications
MG: myasthenia gravis
MHP: moist hot pack
MHz: megahertz
MI: myocardial infarction
MID: multi-infarct dementia
min: minimal
mm: millimeter
mm Hg: millimeters of mercury
MMT: manual muscle test
mod: moderate
MOI: mechanism of injury
mos: months
MRI: magnetic resonance image
MRSA: methicillin-resistant Staphylococcus aureus
MS: multiple sclerosis
MTP: metatarsophalangeal

mV: millivolt
MVA: motor vehicle accident

N or **5/5**: normal (manual muscle test)
N: Newton
n & v: nausea and vomiting
n.: nerve
Na: sodium
N/A: not applicable
n.s.: at bedtime
NBQC: narrow base quad cane
NDT: neurodevelopmental treatment
NICU: neonatal intensive care unit
NIDDM: non-insulin-dependent diabetes mellitus
NIH: National Institutes of Health
NMES: neuromuscular electrical stimulation
NPO: nothing by mouth
NSAID(s): nonsteroidal anti-inflammatory drug(s)
NT: not tested
NWB: non-weightbearing

O: or **"O"**: objective
O2 or O_2: oxygen
OA: osteoarthritis
OASIS: outcome & assessment information set
OB/GYN: obstetrics and gynecology
OBS: organic brain syndrome
OCD: obsessive–compulsive disorder
ODM: opponens digitit minimi
OI: osteogenesis imperfecta
OOB: out of bed
OP: opponens pollicus; outpatient
OR: operating room
ORIF: open reduction internal fixation
OSHA: Occupational Safety & Health Administration
OT: occupational therapist
OTC: over-the-counter (ie, drugs)
OTR/L: occupational therapist registered and licensed
oz: ounce

P or **2/5**: poor (manual muscle test)
p: probability of success
p!: pain
P: or **"P"**: plan
PA: posterior-anterior
PA-C: physician assistant
pc: after meals
PCA: patient-controlled anesthesia
PCL: posterior cruciate ligament
PD: Parkinson's disease
PDR: Physicians' Desk Reference
PE: pulmonary embolism
PEG: percutaneous endoscopic gastrostomy (tube)
PERRLA: pupils equal, round (regular), reactive to light, and accommodating
PET: positron emission tomography
PF: plantarflexion
PFT: pulmonary function test
PI: palmar interossei
PIP: proximal interphalangeal
PL: palmaris longus
PLOF: prior level of function
pm: after noon
PMH: past (or previous) medical history
PNF: proprioceptive neuromuscular facilitation
PNS: peripheral nervous system
po: by mouth
POMR: problem-oriented medical record
post-op: postoperative
PPO: preferred provider organization
PPS: prospective payment system
PQ: pronator quadratus
PRN: as needed
PROM: passive range of motion
PRUJ: proximal radioulnar joint
PT: physical therapist; pronator teres; prothrombin time
Pt. or **pt.**: patient
PTA: physical therapist assistant; prior to admission
PTCA: percutaneous transluminal coronary angioplasty
PTF: posterior talofibular
PTT: partial thromboplastin time
PVD: peripheral vascular disease
PWB: partial weightbearing (usually 50% unless otherwise indicated; may need to check with physician to clarify)

q: every
q2h: every 2 hours
q3h: every 3 hours
q4h: every 4 hours
q8h: every 8 hours
qam: every morning
qh: every hour
qid: 4 times a day
qod: every other day
QS: quad set/quadriceps set

R: or **(R)**: right
RA: rheumatoid arthritis
RBC: red blood cell
RC: radiocarpal
RCL: radial collateral ligament
RD: radial deviation
RDS: respiratory distress syndrome
reps: repetitions
RGO: reciprocating gait orthosis
RHD: right-hand dominant
r/o; **R/O**: rule out
ROM: range of motion
ROS: review of systems
RPE: rate of perceived exertion
RR: respiratory rate

r/s: reschedule
RT: respiratory therapy
RTC: return to clinic
RTW: return to work
RV: residual volume
Rx: prescription

s or **SVN**: supervision
S: or **"S"**: subjective
SAC: short-arm cast
SaO2: oxygen saturation
SAQ: short arc quadriceps exercise
SBA: standby assist
SCI: spinal cord injury
SIDS: sudden infant death syndrome
SL: scapholunate; side lying
SLC: short-leg cast
SLE: systemic lupus erythematosus
SLP: speech language pathologist
SLR: straight-leg raise
SMA: spinal muscular atrophy
SO: shoulder orthosis
SOB: shortness of breath
s/p: status post
SPT: student physical therapist
SPTA: student physical therapist assistant
s/s: signs and/or symptoms
ST: scapulothoracic
stat: immediately
STG: short-term goal
STM: short-term memory
STSG: split-thickness skin graft

T or **1/5**: trace (manual muscle test)
T: temperature
TA: therapeutic activity
TB: tuberculosis
TBI: traumatic brain injury
tbsp or **T**: tablespoon
TFCC: triangular fibrocartilagenous complex
THA: total hip arthroplasty
THR: total hip replacement
TIA: transient ischemic attack
tid: 3 times a day
TKA: total knee arthroplasy
TKE: terminal knee extension
TKR: total knee replacement
TMJ: temporomandibular joint
TP: therapeutic procedure
TPN: total parenteral nutrition
tsp or **t**: teaspoon
TTP: tender to palpation
TTWB: toe-touch weightbearing
TV: tidal volume
tx: traction or treatment

UCL: ulnar collateral ligament
UD: ulnar deviation
UE: upper extremity
UMN: upper motor neuron
US: ultrasound
UTI: urinary tract infection
UV: ultraviolet

V: volt
v/c: verbal cue(s)

W: watt
WBAT: weightbearing as tolerated
WBC: white blood cell
WBQC: wide-base quad cane
w/c: wheelchair
w/cm^2: watts per centimeters squared
WFL: within functional limits
WHFO: wrist-hand-finger orthosis
WHO: wrist-hand orthosis; World Health Organization
wk: week
WNL: within normal limits
WP: whirlpool
WWP: warm whirlpool

y.o.: year old

Common Symbols

about: ~
after: p̄
ascend or **increase**: ↑
at: @
before: ā
degrees Celsius: °C
degrees Fahrenheit: °F
degrees: °
descend or **decrease**: ↓
equal, equal to: (=)
extension: /
female: ♀
flexion: ✓
greater than, greater than or equal to: >, ≥
hour, foot: '
inch, minute: "
less than, less than or **equal to**: <, ≤
male: ♂
micrometer: μ
negative: (–) or –
not equal to, unequal: ≠
number of individuals assisting (one, two): x1, x2
parallel (as in parallel bars): // (// bars)
per: /
positive: (+) or +
possible, question, suggestive: ?

pounds: # or lbs.
primary: 1°
sample mean: x̄
secondary, secondary to: 2°, 2° to
times (as in 3 times per day): x (3x/day)
to/from: ↔
up and down or **ascend and descend**: ↓↑
with: c̄
without: s̄

Index

For Product Safety Concerns and Information please contact our EU representative GPSR@taylorandfrancis.com Taylor & Francis Verlag GmbH, Kaufingerstraße 24, 80331 München, Germany

Printed and bound by CPI Group (UK) Ltd, Croydon, CR0 4YY

08/06/2025

01896981-0006